WITHDRAWN

The
EVERYTHING.
Pregnancy Nutrition Book

Dear Reader:

Congratulations! You have a new bundle of joy on the way! As an expectant mother, you are now undertaking one of the most important roles of your life. Leading a healthy lifestyle now has a whole new meaning. Now more than ever, you need to discover and understand good nutrition and what it will take to properly nourish both you and the baby inside you. Now, more than any other point in your life, is the time to take control of your lifestyle!

Nutrition for yourself can be confusing enough, but now you have another life to consider. At this time in your life there is so much to learn and take in. It can all be so overwhelming. *The Everything® Pregnancy Nutrition Book* will help make one aspect of pregnancy, good nutrition, a bit less confusing and a bit more comprehensible. This book is packed with essential information that you will need both before you become pregnant and during your pregnancy. While this book is a wonderful guide, it is in no way a substitute for the guidance of a qualified health-care provider. Keep in mind that every pregnancy is a unique situation, and this book is only a general guide to your months ahead.

Kimberly A. Tessmer, RD LD

The EVERYTHING® Series

Editorial

Publishing Director	Gary M. Krebs
Managing Editor	Kate McBride
Copy Chief	Laura MacLaughlin
Acquisitions Editor	Kate Burgo
Development Editor	Karen Johnson Jacot
Production Editors	Jamie Wielgus
	Bridget Brace

Production

Production Director	Susan Beale
Production Manager	Michelle Roy Kelly
Series Designers	Daria Perreault
	Colleen Cunningham
	John Paulhus
Cover Design	Paul Beatrice
	Matt LeBlanc
Layout and Graphics	Colleen Cunningham
	Rachael Eiben
	Michelle Roy Kelly
	John Paulhus
	Daria Perreault
	Erin Ring
Series Cover Artist	Barry Littmann
Interior Illustrations	Eulala Connor, Argosy

Visit the entire Everything® Series at www.everything.com

THE
EVERYTHING®
PREGNANCY NUTRITION BOOK

What to eat to ensure a healthy pregnancy

Kimberly A. Tessmer, R.D., L.D.

Adams Media
Avon, Massachusetts

A heartfelt thank you to my incredible husband, Greg Tessmer, who always lends me his unconditional love and support in everything I pursue. To my family and my extraordinary parents, Don and Nancy Bradford, who have always taught me and continuously show me that anything and everything is possible! Thank you to my friends, and a special thank you to a wonderful friend, Megan Jones, for always being there for me and for spurring me on when I needed it the most. I love you all!

An Everything® Series Book.
Everything® and everything.com® are registered trademarks of F+W Publications, Inc.

Published by Adams Media, an F+W Publications Company
57 Littlefield Street, Avon, MA 02322 U.S.A.
www.adamsmedia.com

ISBN: 1-59337-151-9
Printed in the United States of America.

J I H G F E D C B A

Library of Congress Cataloging-in-Publication Data
Tessmer, Kimberly A.
The everything pregnancy nutrition book / Kimberly A. Tessmer.
p.   cm.
An everything series book
ISBN 1-59337-151-9
1. Pregnancy—Nutritional aspects—Popular works. 2. Pregnant women—
Health and hygiene—Popular works. I. Title. II. Series: Everything series.
RG559.T476 2004
618.2'42—dc22
2004013569

This book is available at quantity discounts for bulk purchases.
For information, call 1-800-872-5627.

Contents

Acknowledgments

I am so grateful and indebted to Dr. Alton for all his unique expertise, wonderful ideas, and the time he took out of his very busy schedule to help me create this valuable book. Dr. Alton is an incredible physician with an unbelievable compassion for his patients. I cannot think of a better person or doctor whom I could have asked to assist me. I can't thank you enough! You are the best!!

Top Ten Ways
to Have a Healthier Pregnancy

1. Learn how to eat healthy for two.
2. Know how much of the essential vitamins and minerals you should be getting and why.
3. Learn what foods are safe for you and your baby—and which ones aren't.
4. Understand how total weight gain affects a healthy baby.
5. Learn how to manage the discomforts of pregnancy.
6. Know what to expect though each trimester.
7. Be aware of the special nutritional concerns that can arise during pregnancy.
8. Keep up—or begin—an active lifestyle.
9. Know what drugs and herbal supplements it's okay to take, as well as which ones you should avoid.
10. Understand how particular health conditions may affect your pregnancy.

Introduction
—John A. Alton, M.D.

▶ ONE OF THE MOST difficult aspects of pregnancy is the same one that arises from being a parent: recognizing what is and is not in our control. Life would be so much easier if events in our lives were clearly labeled "in our control" or "not in our control." The most important point to realize is that your nutritional intake during pregnancy plays a vital role in the process. The greatest facet is that nutrition is "Win your control." Fortunately for you, in your hands is a book that explains, clarifies, and updates you on the latest in nutrition and pregnancy. Regardless of whether you just found out you are expecting, are due next week, or are still thinking about starting a family, *The Everything® Pregnancy Nutrition Book* is for you.

Misinformation causes confusion, which can result in wasted energy, worry, and possibly harmful habits. Some of the greatest advances in science over the last few decades are in the area of nutrition. The education of the individual regarding these changes is very exciting. To understand how greatly our diet impacts not only our health but also that of our unborn child makes us thirst for even more knowledge. Many of my patients are very aware of small changes in their bodies, and they take cues from their bodies to change their lifestyles. In pregnancy, those cues can be misleading. Therefore, a guide such as this book will help you through the one area in your control—your diet and lifestyle.

Unfortunately, our society holds that attitude that good parenting is something that comes naturally, and unfortunately that falsehood starts with pregnancy. This misinformation usually is not from books that are written by experienced professionals but from friends, acquaintances, family, or past experiences. Every pregnancy is as unique as the child that is born. Listen to others' opinions, find out their sources, and then verify the information. This book is a great resource for verification. When we purchase our new cars, televisions, or cell phones, we look at the owner's manual to learn about features, maintenance, or troubleshooting. Think of this book as your owner's manual to pregnancy.

Make this book a companion to your prenatal visits and read it in the waiting room. By reading this book and taking notes in the margins or listing questions for your doctor or midwife, you will be better prepared to make the most of those visits. When patients bring a list of questions, it shows they are taking the time be active participants in their pregnancies. The supporting partner, whether it is a spouse, relative, or friend of the expectant mother, will also find this book an informative reference for the forty weeks of pregnancy. Almost as important, they will find this information handy during the time before pregnancy occurs. So often we want to help those we care for but are unsure how to be effective. By reading this book, and gaining knowledge, the partner can be more supporting and play a more intimate and special role in the pregnancy.

Be aware that no matter how well you listen to your doctor or midwife or follow the guidelines in the book, unfortunate events can happen that are beyond anyone's control. To assign blame and look for an answer as to why it happened is normal human nature. But if you take the time to read this book, you will have done everything in your control to give your unborn child the best start he or she could have. After all, that is what everyone wants.

Consider this book and your pregnancy as a springboard to a healthier lifestyle for you and your family. This book is the first step in impacting the one area of your pregnancy that is within your control. The information and confidence you will gain will change the rest of your life.

Chapter 1

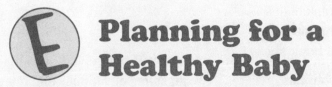 **Planning for a Healthy Baby**

If you are planning to have a baby, consuming an ideal diet and living a healthy lifestyle are extremely important. What you do before pregnancy can have a large impact on the outcome of your pregnancy. A well-planned, nutritious diet that includes the right balance of essential nutrients is the first step you should take in planning for a healthy baby.

Healthy Eating for Your Baby

Eating healthily will ensure that both you and your fetus receive the nutrients that are essential for you both from the very start of pregnancy. But don't wait until you are pregnant. Researchers believe that eating a healthy diet once you become pregnant may not make up for earlier nutritional deficiencies.

Supplying Nutrients for Your Baby

In the very first weeks of pregnancy, often before you even realize you are pregnant, your baby will rely on your stores of vitamins and minerals for normal development. During pregnancy, optimal nutrition will be in high demand. Your body needs enough nutrients to support itself, as well as the baby, through all stages of development. All the nourishment your baby needs will come from the foods you eat, the reserves in your body, and the supplements that you take. The key to a healthy birth is to start eating a healthy diet and boosting your intake of certain essential nutrients before you become pregnant. It's all about planning ahead! You plan for the baby's room and for the supplies and clothes you need, and so on. Don't forget the most important plan—a healthy you!

To begin, you need to ask yourself whether your eating habits measure up and whether you are getting the nutrients you need to support a healthy pregnancy. If the answer is "no," you have some work to do. Start by assessing your present eating habits. A good assessment tool is the USDA's Food Guide Pyramid. Keep in mind that it is important to get your partner started on a healthier lifestyle, too.

Assessing Your Diet with the Food Guide Pyramid

The Food Guide Pyramid can be used as a tool to assess your current food intake. The pyramid contains all the food groups essential to a healthy diet. It is meant as a guideline to aid people in recognizing what and how much to eat of each of the five major food groups daily. Following the Food Guide Pyramid will help keep your fat intake at healthy levels and ensure that you are consuming all the essential nutrients that make up a healthy diet for the average person. It will help you increase your intake of nutrient-dense foods or foods that contain more nutrients than calories. By following the Food Guide Pyramid, you can rest assured that you are getting all of the nourishment that your body needs to plan for a healthy pregnancy.

FIGURE 1-1
The USDA Food
Guide Pyramid

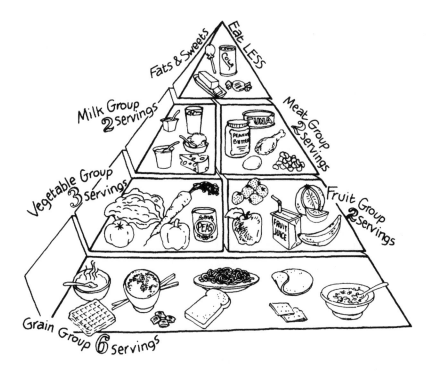

Source: U.S. Department of Agriculture and the U.S. Department of Health and Human Services.

On average, women who are not pregnant should consume the following servings daily from the Food Guide Pyramid (depending on activity level):

- 6 to 9 servings from the bread, cereal, rice, and pasta group—Include whole-grain and whole-wheat foods as much as possible.
- 3 to 4 servings from the vegetable group—Choose from a variety of vegetables, and stick to fresh or frozen for higher nutritional content.
- 2 to 3 servings from the fruit group—Choose from a variety of fruits.
- 2 to 3 servings from the milk group—Choose from low-fat or fat-free dairy products.

- 5 to 6 ounces (or 2 servings) from the meat group—Choose from lean meats and include nonmeat protein foods such as beans, lentils, and fish regularly.
- Fats, oils, and sweets—Use sparingly.

Keep in mind that the stated number of servings is for women who are not yet pregnant. These serving sizes increase with pregnancy and are discussed in more detail in Chapter 3.

Food in one group should not replace foods from another group. Because each group supplies different essential nutrients, no food group is any more important than any other. It is important to eat from all of the food groups each day and to eat a variety for optimal nutritional intake. In addition to your food intake, don't forget your fluids, too!

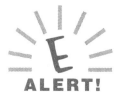

ALERT!

Water is an important nutrient and one that is often overlooked when planning a healthy diet. For optimal intake, you should shoot for at least eight 8-ounce glasses per day. Water is present in just about every part of the body and has a vital role in almost every major function in the body, including pregnancy. The body has no provision to store water, so make sure you drink water every day.

Principles of Healthy Eating

The Dietary Guidelines for Americans are made up of ten basic principles for healthy eating. The guidelines are meant to provide sound advice to help people make food choices for a healthy, active life. Following the guidelines will ensure that your eating habits measure up. Therefore, understanding the dietary guidelines should be your first step to making sure you are consuming a diet that is optimal to a healthy pregnancy.

The Dietary Guidelines for Americans

The dietary guidelines follow an easy-to-remember "ABC" organization. Each of the three main topics (Aim for Fitness, Build a Healthy Base, and Choose Sensibly) includes several important points. (To read the full guidelines, see Appendix A.)

The first topic, Aim for Fitness, points out the important of good physical health:

- Aim for a healthy weight.
- Be physically active each day.

The second topic, Build a Healthy Base, gives basic pointers on healthy eating:

- Let the pyramid guide your food choices.
- Choose a variety of grains daily, especially whole grains.
- Choose a variety of fruits and vegetables daily.
- Keep food safe to eat.

The third topic, Choose Sensibly, provides advice on eating for general health:

- Choose a diet that is low in saturated fat and cholesterol and moderate in total fat.
- Choose beverages and foods to moderate your intake of sugars.
- Choose and prepare foods with less salt.
- If you drink alcoholic beverages, do so in moderation.

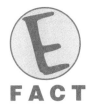

The Dietary Guidelines for Americans are published by the U.S. Department of Agriculture (USDA) and the U.S. Department of Health and Human Services. The guidelines are updated every five years. To be on the cutting edge of good health, look for updated versions as they become available.

Changing Your Eating Habits

Let's say that after a review of the Food Guide Pyramid and the USDA's dietary guidelines, you have determined that your nutritional intake in not up to par. Don't worry—there is time to make some changes. The key is to make only a few changes at a time. Trying to change your entire diet at one time can be frustrating and discouraging. Start with simple goals—such as eating at least three meals a day, eating two servings of fruit per day, drinking eight glasses of water each day, or walking thirty minutes three times per week—and work your way up from there. Once you have mastered one set of habits, move on to the next. Be sure your goals are realistic, specific, and attainable. "Eat more fruit" is a noble goal, but it might help to make one that's more specific, like goal is "Eat two servings of fruit each day."

To aid in your endeavors, find a way to monitor yourself, such as a food journal. Self-monitoring has been shown to help change a behavior in the desired direction. Keep in mind that it takes at least twenty-one days to actually change a habit—be patient. Use your food journal to write down everything you eat and drink throughout the day; this can help you stay committed to your goals of eating a healthier diet. Write each item down as soon as you have eaten it. That way you won't conveniently forget to take note of certain foods at the end of the day. Keep track of your exercise habits and how much water you drink, too.

Before You Become Pregnant

There are several dietary guidelines that everyone should follow, but there are also specific guidelines for women who are planning to become pregnant. In the months before a woman becomes pregnant, her nutritional intake can be a key factor in the outcome of the pregnancy. The foods she eats and the vitamins and minerals she takes will help ensure that both she and the fetus have the nutrients required right from the very start of the pregnancy.

General Pre-Pregnancy Tips

The key to a healthy pregnancy diet is to plan ahead. First, work to improve your diet. You, as well as your partner, need to follow a well-balanced healthy diet with at least three meals per day. Meals should be spaced evenly throughout the day and should provide foods from all of the food groups. If you are not sure how to go about eating healthier, now is the perfect time to make an appointment with a registered dietitian who can point you in the right direction.

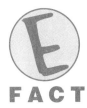

FACT

Most of a baby's major organs form very early in pregnancy. Birth defects and other problems can occur before a woman has missed her first period or knows she is pregnant. You can lower the risk of birth defects and problems with pregnancy by making healthy nutritional choices before you even get pregnant.

Make a prenatal doctor's visit, and get a checkup before you become pregnant. This will ensure you are in good health. If you have medical problems, an early visit to your doctor can help get your problem under control and can give you a heads-up for what you might need to do or expect during pregnancy. Talk to your doctor about your family history, including genetics and birth defects. While at your doctor, ask about beginning a prenatal supplement to ensure you are getting all of the nutrients you need. These supplements can help build up the nutritional stores that can be depleted quickly during pregnancy. They can also ensure you are getting essential nutrients, such as folic acid, that help prevent birth defects.

Reaching a healthy weight may mean losing or gaining weight before trying to conceive. Make sure that you are at a healthy weight or working toward it. The body mass index (BMI) is one tool that can be used to determine a healthy weight. You should use the BMI only as a general guide. Many factors need to be considered when estimating how much a person should weigh. See Appendix B for information on figuring your BMI.

Get yourself on a regular exercise plan. Being in good physical shape at least three months or more before you conceive can make it easier to maintain an active lifestyle while you are pregnant. It can also be a benefit during labor. Physical fitness can help maintain good moods and energy levels as well as get you back in shape quicker after you deliver. Part of fitness is the ability to cope well with daily challenges. Do what you can to reduce your stress levels, and learn to cope with your stress through meditation, exercise or other coping methods.

Take a look at your lifestyle habits, and begin to make changes to bad habits. Research shows that smoking, drinking, and taking drugs are most definitely connected to low birth-weight babies, miscarriages, sudden infant-death syndrome (SIDS), and possible behavioral problems later in life. It is best to stop these habits before trying to have a baby.

Avoid using hazardous substances and chemicals, including many household cleaning products. Be careful about what products you use and how.

Do what you can to take care of yourself and avoid infections. Some infections can be harmful to the fetus, so keep up your resistance. You can do this by washing your hands, keeping your distance from people around you who are sick, and staying away from unsafe foods.

Nutritional Needs for All Women

Your first plan of action should be to ensure that you are receiving all of the nutrients needed for optimal health in your age range. Some nutrient needs, as well as calorie needs, will increase with pregnancy and breast-feeding. But your increased need for vitamins and minerals is immediate and does not depend on whether you are pregnant. Vitamins and minerals are key nutrients to every process that takes place in your body. They work together to make all your body processes happen normally. Your needs for certain nutrients are more imperative before and during pregnancy. Specific nutrients that are important include folate, calcium, and iron.

The Dangers of Mega-Dosing

Just because a vitamin or mineral is beneficial, more does not always mean better. Some vitamins and minerals have toxic effects at very high levels; for instance, be particularly aware of your intake of iodine and vitamins A, D, E, and K. Let's take the example of vitamin A to see how high levels can be ingested and a sample potential danger of ingesting too much of a nutrient. Other vitamins and minerals in too-high doses carry different risks; pay attention to what you eat, and be sure to go to your doctor with any questions or concerns.

Vitamin A is important for promoting the growth and health of cells and tissues in both the mother and fetus. Vitamin A needs are not increased during pregnancy because the reserves in a woman's body easily meet the needs of the fetus. In fact, research suggests that excess vitamin A ingested from supplements—over 10,000 international units (IU) daily—can be toxic and increase the risk of birth defects. Vitamin A in larger amounts poses the most risk two weeks prior to conception and during the first two months of pregnancy. These findings do not pertain to beta-carotene, a precursor of vitamin A, which does not pose a risk and is not toxic. Check any supplements you take to learn the source of the vitamin A, and take in this vitamin only in amounts recommended or prescribed by your doctor. Stay away from mega doses of any vitamin or mineral before, during, and after pregnancy.

Focus on Folic Acid

Folate, found naturally in foods, is one of the B vitamins; it is also known as folic acid, which is the name for the form found in supplements and fortified foods. Folic acid merits special consideration. During pregnancy, this vitamin helps to properly develop the neural tube, which becomes the baby's spine. When taken in daily optimal amounts at least one month before becoming pregnant and during the first trimester, folic acid can help prevent birth defects of the brain and spinal cord, called neural tube defects (NTDs).

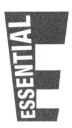

Though the Instutite of Medicine of the National Acadamies still states that the recommended intake is 400 mcg for women of childbearing age, recent studies show that to decrease the risk of birth defects, folic acid should be increased to 800 to 1000 mcg daily (the amount in most prenatal vitamins) in those attempting pregnancy. So your doctor will likely prescribe a prenatal vitamin with this higher amount.

Spina bifida, sometimes called "open spine," affects the backbone and sometimes the spinal cord. Spina bifida is the most common severe birth defect in the United States, affecting 1,500 to 2,000 babies (1 in every 2,000 live births) each year. Anencephaly is a fatal condition in which the baby is born with a severely underdeveloped brain and skull.

Because most women do not know that they are pregnant right away and because the neural tube and the brain begin to form so quickly after conception, taking optimal amounts of folic acid on a daily basis is important for all women in their childbearing years.

Intake Requirements

Even though a woman follows a healthy, well-balanced diet, she may still not be consuming the recommended amount of folic acid each day. For this reason, in 1998 the Institute of Medicine recommended "that to reduce their risk for an NTD-affected pregnancy, women capable of becoming pregnant should take at least 400 mcg of synthetic folic acid daily, from fortified foods or supplements or a combination of the two, in addition to consuming food folate from a varied diet." You can use an over-the-counter multivitamin/mineral supplement or prenatal supplement to make sure you get your folic acid. Check the label on over-the-counter supplements because not all contain folic acid in the recommended amounts. The intake for folate increases with pregnancy and breastfeeding. Women who have previously had a baby with an NTD may have higher folate requirements and should speak with their doctors.

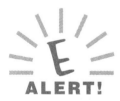

ALERT!

Until more information becomes available, both pregnant and non-pregnant women ages nineteen years and older should not exceed the tolerable upper limit of 1,000 mcg of folate per day from foods, fortified foods, and supplements unless otherwise prescribed by their doctor.

To help women consume more folate, in 1998 the U.S. Food and Drug Administration (FDA) required that all grain products such as breads, flour, crackers, and rice be fortified with folic acid. Other very good sources of folate include orange juice, fortified breakfast cereals, lentils, dried beans, dark-green leafy vegetables, spinach, broccoli, peanuts, wheat germ, and avocados. Folate can be destroyed during cooking, so eat fruits and vegetables raw or cook them for as short a time as possible by steaming, microwaving, or stir-frying.

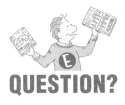

QUESTION?

Do folic acid supplements really make that much of a difference in preventing certain birth defects?
According to the U.S. Centers for Disease Control (CDC), when taken one month before conception and throughout the first trimester, folic acid supplements have been proven to reduce the risk for an NTD-affected pregnancy by 50 to 70 percent.

Charge Up the Calcium

Calcium is a mineral that deserves special attention throughout a woman's life, especially when it comes to pregnancy. Calcium is important to strong bones and teeth, a healthy heart, nerves, and muscles, and the development of normal heart rhythm and blood-clotting abilities. Not consuming enough calcium and/or not having good calcium stores will force the baby to use calcium from your own bones. Consuming plenty of calcium before, during, and after pregnancy can also help to reduce your risk for osteoporosis, or brittle bone disease, later in life.

Intake Requirements

Whether pregnant or not, calcium needs for teens (age fourteen to eighteen) is 1,300 milligrams (mg) and 1,000 mg for woman nineteen to fifty. Women older than fifty need 1,200 mg of calcium daily. The tolerable upper intake level for calcium is 2,500 mg daily.

The easiest way to get all the calcium you need is to eat at least two to three servings of low-fat or fat-free dairy foods each day. Other sources include green leafy vegetables, calcium-fortified orange juice, calcium-fortified soy milk, fish with edible bones, and tofu made with calcium sulfate. Reading the nutrition facts panel (included on all packaged foods) is a great way to spot calcium-rich foods. The amount on the panel is presented in terms of "% Daily Value," which is an approximation of the percentage of your day's calcium need supplied by one serving of that food.

Most prenatal supplements do not provide all of the calcium you need daily. You may need to take a calcium supplement, especially if you are not a milk drinker, are a strict vegetarian, or are lactose intolerant. There are all types of calcium supplements on the market today. Ideally, a calcium supplement should also contain vitamin D for maximum absorption to occur.

Elemental Calcium

In a discussion of the amount of calcium in supplements, it is important to understand the concept of elemental calcium. Calcium occurs in combination with other substances, forming compounds such as calcium carbonate, calcium phosphate, or calcium citrate. What is really important is the "elemental" calcium, or the actual amount of calcium in the compound. Some compounds contain more elemental calcium than others. For instance, a calcium supplement made from calcium carbonate might have 625 mg in each tablet, but the amount of elemental calcium in each tablet is about 250 mg. When looking for a calcium supplement, be sure to read the label carefully. Ideally, the label will list how much elemental calcium is in each tablet. If the label does not state elemental calcium, you can figure it out with the following chart. Elemental calcium accounts for these percentages of the following compounds:

- 40 percent of calcium carbonate
- 21 percent of calcium citrate
- 13 percent of calcium lactate
- 9 percent of calcium gluconate

How to Take Calcium Supplements

Supplements that contain calcium citrate can be taken with or without food, whereas calcium carbonate should be taken with food for optimal absorption. Many antacids, such as Tums, contain calcium carbonate, which may be a more convenient and less expensive way to take your calcium. If you prefer a chewable pill, products such as Viactiv can be a good choice. Avoid the natural-source calcium pills, such as those produced from oyster shell, dolomite, or bone meal. These supplements may contain lead or other toxic metals. When taking calcium supplements, it is best to take smaller amounts several times a day for the best absorption. If you are taking a calcium supplement and an iron supplement or a supplement with iron in it, take them at different times of the day. They will each be better absorbed alone.

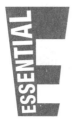

Regular exercise can have many healthy benefits for pregnant women, including making the birthing process easier. It is a good idea to start an exercise program before you become pregnant. This will give you time to adjust and will help get your body ready for pregnancy. Women who are already exercising before pregnancy can continue to do so, but they may need to decrease the intensity. Women who are not exercising before pregnancy can start, but they must start very slowly and should consult their doctor first. Talk to your doctor about the amount of exercise that is safe for you.

Pump Up the Iron

Iron is another essential mineral that merits special attention as part of your diet before and during pregnancy. Iron is essential to the formation of healthy red blood cells, which are responsible for carrying oxygen through your blood to the cells of your body. Almost two-thirds of the iron in your body is found in hemoglobin, the protein in red blood cells that carries oxygen to your body's tissues. The increase in blood volume that takes place during pregnancy greatly increases a woman's need for iron. If you do not get enough iron and/or do not have adequate iron stores, the growing baby will take it at your expense. Iron deficiency during pregnancy can cause anemia, extreme fatigue, a low birth-weight baby, and other potential problems. The greater your iron stores before you become pregnant, the better iron will be absorbed during pregnancy.

Intake Requirements

It is very difficult to get enough iron from foods alone. Most multi-vitamin/mineral supplements and/or prenatal vitamin supplements will provide you with your pre-pregnancy needs of 18 mg per day. If you have anemia before becoming pregnant, your doctor may prescribe a much larger dose. During pregnancy, your iron requirement climbs to 27 mg per day.

Again, as with many other vitamin and minerals, too much iron is not always best. Iron has a tolerable upper intake level of 45 mg. Foods that supply iron include meat, poultry, fish, legumes, and whole-grain and enriched grain products. Iron from plant sources (or "nonheme iron") is not as easily absorbed as that from animal sources (or "heme iron"). Supplementing your meals with a food or beverage rich in vitamin C, such as citrus fruits or juices, broccoli, tomatoes, or kiwi, will help your body better absorb the iron in the foods you consume. The absorption of iron from supplements is best absorbed on an empty stomach or when swallowed with juice containing vitamin C.

The Scoop on Prenatal Vitamins

Prenatal supplements (PNVs) are specialized vitamin and mineral supplements that women can take even before pregnancy to get all of the essential nutrients they need during pregnancy. Studies have shown that the use of prenatal supplements before and throughout pregnancy can benefit a healthy baby.

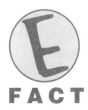

FACT

Vitamins and minerals should never replace a healthy diet. They are only meant to supplement a healthy diet, not take the place of any one food or any food group. Foods contain hundreds of vitamins, minerals, and phytonutrients. Only food supplies the ideal mixture of these substances that are essential for optimal health. Supplements can provide you with insurance that you will receive everything you need, but they cannot do the entire job.

Prenatal vitamins come in many formulations. Most PNV are distributed as samples to physician's offices, and it is a good idea to try multiple samples because some have stool softeners and other binders, which you may or may not tolerate. Finding one that you can tolerate will make it easier to take and therefore easier to remember to take it daily.

The Ideal Prenatal Vitamin

The components all PNV supplements should have in common are folic acid, iron, and calcium. Most PNVs have only 100 to 250 mg of calcium—women need 1,000 to 1,200 mg daily, so you should also take a separate calcium supplement. Except for calcium, you should never take any additional supplements with your prenatal supplement unless they are prescribed by your doctor. Since some over-the-counter supplements contain too-high levels of vitamins and minerals, it may be smarter to use a supplement such as a PNV that has been specifically formulated for pregnant women and/or women trying to conceive. PNVs are not recommended postpartum unless the mother is considered to be at "nutritional risk." Some women can benefit from taking prenatal vitamins postpartum if they plan to become pregnant in less than one year, but most experts recommend spacing pregnancy by at least one year.

Who Should Take Supplements?

If you are a healthy woman who eats a well-balanced diet and has no risk factors, your doctor may not feel that you need to take a prenatal supplement. This is something that you need to discuss with your doctor so together you can determine what is right for you. No matter how healthily you eat, it is generally difficult to get what you need each and every day, especially while pregnant or trying to conceive, so a prenatal supplement can act as insurance. All doctors do agree that a folic acid supplement is necessary.

Women who have a history of poor eating habits, who are on a restricted diet such as a vegan diet, or who require a specific nutrient due to an existing medical condition will definitely need to take some type of supplement.

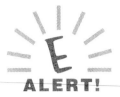

ALERT!

Women who are expecting more than one baby or have closely spaced pregnancies will need extra iron and may require additional vitamin and mineral supplementation. Nourishing two babies demands more from your body and therefore requires more nutrients. After pregnancy, your body may be depleted of some nutrients. If you are planning to become pregnant again soon, you may need special supplements to restore those nutrients. Speak to your doctor before starting any supplement program.

Are Your Prenatals Making You Sick?

Many women have trouble taking prenatal vitamins once they become pregnant because the iron content can exacerbate morning sickness. They are also known to cause constipation and gas. If you are having problems, try taking your prenatal vitamins with food or taking them right before bedtime. Also drink plenty of water and include plenty of fiber in your diet. If that doesn't work, talk to your doctor about trying a different brand or switching to a prenatal supplement without iron for the first trimester. Many times these problems only last for the first trimester. In the meantime, make certain your prenatal contains vitamin B_6. This vitamin has been found to help relieve nausea in some women during pregnancy, a common discomfort during the first trimester.

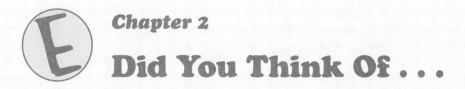

Chapter 2

Did You Think Of . . .

You now have your nutritional intake on track, but there are plenty of other factors to consider before you become pregnant. You have a lot to think about, including your health-care provider, fertility, lifestyle changes, current health problems, and family history. Planning ahead and being prepared can be the formula for a less complicated and safer pregnancy.

Your Prenatal Care

Ideally, your prenatal care should begin before you even become pregnant. According to the U.S. Centers for Disease Control and Prevention, almost 4 million American women give birth each year. Nearly one-third of them will experience some type of pregnancy-related complication. Women who do not seek adequate prenatal care increase their risk for complications that may go undetected or are not dealt with soon enough. This can lead to serious consequences for the mother and/or baby. It's never too early to start prenatal care.

Your doctor can do a thorough physical exam and can explain how pregnancy might affect you as an individual. Your doctor can address any current health issues you may have and discuss with you how it may affect your pregnancy. She can review any medications you are taking and make any changes necessary. She can also make sure you are up to date on immunizations, test you for HIV and other sexually transmitted diseases, and measure your immunity to certain childhood diseases such as chicken pox and rubella. It is a smart idea to have these tests done before you get pregnant to make sure you are in good health. Your prenatal check up is also your chance to ask any questions you may have.

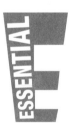

If you follow a strict vegetarian diet or participate in strenuous exercise such as long-distance running, your levels of key nutrients and hormones may be affected. Prescription medications, weight-loss diets, anemia, and other health issues also affect these levels, so you should talk to your doctor before trying to get pregnant.

Choosing a Health-Care Provider

Choosing your health-care provider—and the hospital where you'll have your baby—can be one of the most important decisions you make for you and your baby. Women who are planning to become pregnant are typically cared for by either a board-certified obstetrician/gynecologist (OB/GYN), a family practitioner, or a certified nurse-midwife (CNM). Your health-care provider might be your current OB/GYN or family doctor (if he specializes in obstetrics), or you may want to take this chance to switch doctors if you are not completely comfortable with your present one. Choose a health-care professional who is caring enough to spend a few extra minutes with you to talk about preconception care. The recommendation of family members, friends, and insurance companies can be helpful as well.

Demystifying the Titles

Obstetricians (OB) are doctors who specialize in pregnancy and childbirth. These doctors may or may not also be gynecologists (GYN), who are doctors specializing in women's health care. If your doctor is board certified, you will see the letters FACOG (Fellow of the American College of Obstetricians and Gynecologists) following her name.

A certified nurse midwife (CNM) is an advanced practice nurse who specializes in women's health care, including prenatal care, labor, and delivery, and postpartum care for "normal" pregnancies. Most midwives in the United States are CNMs. They have at least a bachelor's degree, and some may have a master's or doctoral degree. Certification means the nurse midwife has completed both nursing and midwifery training and has passed national and state licensing exams to become certified. Midwives are now licensed to practice in all states, and many work in conjunction with doctors. About 96 percent of CNM-assisted births occur in hospitals. Certified midwives are not registered nurses, but otherwise they meet the same qualifications as a CNM. Currently, only the State of New York recognizes this certification as sufficient for licensure. If you choose a midwife to perform the delivery, make sure to ask about that midwife's credentialing process. Also find out who is supervising her in your care and the delivery of your baby.

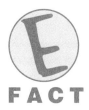

FACT

CNM-attended births are becoming much more popular. In fact, the American College of Nurse-Midwives estimates that from 1989 to 2000, the number of CNM-attended births increased by almost 125 percent.

It is up to you to make an educated and informed decision about who will care for you and your baby during pregnancy, so do your research. If you are considered higher risk due to your personal health and/or personal or family health history or there is reason to anticipate complications during your pregnancy or childbirth, you may need to choose a doctor who specializes in your condition. Your OB/GYN should be able to help you pinpoint risk factors and refer you to a specialist if necessary. No matter whom you choose, it is important to make your decision and make a prenatal appointment as soon as possible.

Fertility and Nutrition

Do you want to create your best chance for becoming pregnant? For both women and men, there is a definite link between nutrition and fertility. Sticking with a well-balanced diet boosts your chances of getting pregnant and having a healthy baby. You should begin making changes to your eating habits at least three months to a year before planning to get pregnant.

Certain vitamins and minerals, such as vitamins C and E and zinc and folic acid, are crucial for creating healthy sperm. Several studies have indicated that deficiencies in zinc can impede both female and male fertility. You should maintain the dietary reference intake (DRI) of 8 mg per day for women over eighteen years and 11 mg per day for men over eighteen to help keep your reproductive system functioning properly. Men who are deficient in folate have been shown to experience a lower number and poorer quality of sperm. Being deficient in certain nutrients may affect a woman's menstrual periods, which makes it more difficult to predict when she is ovulating and the best time for her to get pregnant. Maintaining a diet that includes all of the food groups and living a healthier lifestyle will ensure the most favorable reproductive functioning.

Herbs have also been used for many years to treat all types of health conditions. Today, herbs are even becoming popular as fertility enhancers, and it never hurts to research all of your options. You should always seek the advice of your health-care provider before taking any new supplement, regardless of whether it is "natural" or not. Many health-care professionals are hesitant about herbs, which are not currently regulated by the FDA or the scrutiny of clinical studies, while prescription medications are. In addition, many factors can affect their potency. Some of the most popular herbs used for promoting fertility include vitex angus, black cohosh, dong quai, licorice, Korean ginseng, and pycnogenol.

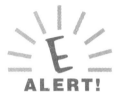

ALERT!

You should never mix herbs with prescription fertility drugs. Herbs can also interact with other prescription medications, so always speak to your doctor before starting any program that includes herbs. All herbs should be discontinued once you find out you are pregnant.

Keep in mind that some herbs on the market can actually decrease fertility. St. John's Wort, for instance, can decrease sperm motility in men. Do your research and speak with your doctor before taking any herbal supplement.

Kicking Your Habits

Not only is it vital to a healthier lifestyle—not to mention a healthy pregnancy and a healthy baby—to kick some bad habits, evidence shows that kicking bad habits such as alcohol, smoking, drug use, and caffeine can also increase chances for conceiving. You should begin to make these healthier lifestyle changes at least three months to a year before you plan to conceive. When it comes to fertility, a healthy lifestyle is just as important for men as for women. Sperm can be affected by alcohol, tobacco, drug use, and caffeine as much as a woman's eggs. Some research suggests that certain bad habits can contribute to lower sperm counts and slower sperm motility.

Alcohol

Drinking alcohol during pregnancy can cause both mental and physical birth defects in babies and may result in deformities, social or learning problems, and sometimes death. There is no safe level of alcohol during pregnancy, and it should be completely avoided. That includes the time you are trying to conceive, since many times you may be pregnant before you realize it. According to recent studies, women who drink alcohol while trying to conceive, even in small amounts, may reduce their chances of becoming pregnant. Alcohol-related birth defects are more likely to result from the intake of alcohol during the first trimester, when the brain and many of the baby's organs are developing. Growth problems are likely to result from drinking alcohol in the third trimester. Drinking at any stage of the pregnancy can affect the brain. Drinking alcohol can also increase the risk of miscarriage, low birth weight, and stillbirth babies as well as fetal alcohol syndrome. If you are having a problem with not drinking, you should seek professional help.

Tobacco

Cigarette smoking or any other kind of tobacco use can be very hazardous throughout your pregnancy. Smoking has been proven to cause miscarriages and preterm delivery, as well as infant death. Smoking can cause low birth weight, asthma in infants and young children, SIDS, and other respiratory diseases. People who smoke inhale nicotine and carbon monoxide, both of which can travel through the placenta directly to the baby. This can prevent the fetus from receiving the oxygen and the nutrients it needs to grow and develop properly. Secondhand smoke can be just as hazardous and should be avoided when possible. After pregnancy, it is important to remember that your breast milk often contains what is in your body. If you smoke while breastfeeding, your baby can ingest the nicotine in your milk.

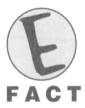

FACT

According to the American Lung Association, "Smoking during pregnancy accounts for an estimated 20 to 30 percent of low birth-weight babies, up to 14 percent of preterm deliveries, and some 10 percent of all infant deaths."

It will not protect your baby if you merely cut down on your smoking or switch to lower tar cigarettes. Women must quit smoking while trying to conceive, while pregnant, and while breastfeeding. This can be the perfect time to stop smoking for life and help decrease your risk of developing future tobacco-related health problems, such as cancer and heart disease.

Kicking the habit can take time, so get started well before you begin trying to conceive.

Caffeine

The risk of caffeine intake during pregnancy is a controversial issue. Still, most experts agree that you should cut back on your caffeine consumption while trying to conceive and while you are pregnant. That doesn't mean you have to completely cut out caffeine, but you should cut down. Most research shows that it is safe to drink coffee or other caffeinated beverages during pregnancy as long as you consume less than three cups, or about 300 mg of caffeine per day (per the American Dietetic Association). Consumption of more than 300 mg per day has been associated with a possible decrease in fertility and an increase risk of miscarriage or low birth-weight babies.

Caffeine acts as a mild stimulant to the central nervous system and also has a diuretic effect, which increases water loss from the body through urination. Neither of these effects is favorable during pregnancy or even for good health in general. Caffeine can also decrease the amount of calcium your body absorbs and can increase loss of calcium through the urine. This effect of caffeine becomes more prominent if dietary calcium intake is already inadequate. Many over-the-counter pain relievers, cold medications, allergy medications, and diet pills contain as much caffeine as a cup or two of coffee, so read labels carefully. When purchasing over-the-counter medications, ask the pharmacist which are best. Be sure to mention that you are pregnant or trying to cut down on your caffeine intake. Many energy drinks on the market today also contain very high levels of caffeine.

While many doctors recommend cutting back on caffeine, others recommend cutting it out of your diet completely, especially if you are in a high-risk category. Some doctors may recommend cutting out caffeine completely during the first trimester and then restricting amounts during the remainder of the pregnancy. Talk with your doctor about your best options. Decaffeinated beverages are fine, but be sure they are not crowding out more nutritious beverages such as milk, water, and juice. When in doubt, do without!

If you are a caffeine junkie, cutting back or cutting out caffeine can be difficult and may cause headaches and fatigue. Cut back gradually, and work to have it under control by the time you are ready to conceive.

Drug Use

It is crucial that while trying to conceive, women and their partners avoid recreational drugs such as marijuana, cocaine, and other illegal drugs, and it is especially important for the mother to avoid them during pregnancy and breastfeeding. Many recreational drugs are highly addictive, and users may need professional help to kick the habit for good. Most of these drugs can reach the fetus by crossing the placenta and can also be passed through breast milk.

Studies show that using marijuana during pregnancy can result in low birth weight, malformations, poor growth, and fetal neurological problems. The male sperm can also be affected by using this drug. It can take one month for the drug to be completely out of the body, so a woman should quit using any drugs at least a month before even trying to conceive.

The message is simple: If you want to have a healthy baby and a healthy pregnancy, illicit recreational drugs have no place in your lifestyle. These drugs have no place in the environment of an infant, and the time to kick these habits is before you even attempt to conceive. Be honest with your doctor—if you are a user, let him know so that you can get the help that you need.

Your Pre-Pregnancy Weight

Being either overweight or underweight before and during pregnancy can cause problems. Before pregnancy, being significantly over- or underweight has been shown to interfere with ovulation and fertility. Your goal should be to reach a healthy weight or be as close as possible before you conceive. Being overweight can increase your risk for high blood pressure and gestational diabetes as well as increase the risk of some birth defects. Researchers from the U.S. Centers for Disease Control and Prevention have found a link between pre-pregnancy obesity and the increased risk of neural tube birth defects, including spina bifida. Being overweight but not obese at the time of conception resulted in increased risks of having a child with heart defects or more than one unrelated birth defect. Underweight women increase the risk of having a low birth-weight baby and a premature delivery. If a woman is underweight due to undereating, she may not be supplying her body with all the nutrients she needs for a healthy baby.

What Is a Healthy Weight?

A healthy weight is a realistic weight that is best for you—not necessarily the lowest weight you *think* you should be or the "ideal weight" you feel you should be. People come in all shapes and sizes, so it is impossible to use ideal weights or talk about what a "perfect" body should be. A healthy weight is one that puts you at the least risk for health problems related to your weight. The following chart can give you a general idea of whether you are at a healthy weight.

FIGURE 2-1

Healthy Weight Chart

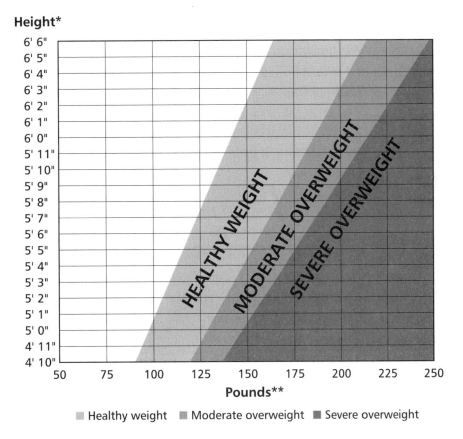

* Without shoes.

** Without clothes. The higher weights apply to people with more muscle and bone, such as many men.

Source: Report of the Dietary Guidelines Advisory Committee on the *Dietary Guidelines for Americans,* 1995, pp. 23–24.

Another tool to help evaluate your weight is the body mass index (BMI), which calculates what percentage of your weight is body fat. You can find the formula for calculating your BMI in Appendix B.

Not At a Healthy Weight?

If you are not at a healthy weight, it is time to think about how you will get there before you begin trying to conceive. Eating to control your weight and eating for good health are really one and the same. A healthy diet and regular exercise can accomplish both goals. To lose weight, you simply need to eat fewer healthy calories, and for weight gain you need to eat more.

If you are overweight, a safe and healthy weight loss is a deficit of 250 to 1,000 calories per day to lose ½ pound to 2 pounds per week. Losing weight any quicker than that means you are losing muscle mass instead of body fat. To lose 1 pound of fat, you need to burn 3,500 more calories than you take in. In other words, losing 1 pound of fat per week means taking in 500 fewer calories per day from your maintenance diet.

Your main goal should be to lose weight safely and sensibly. Therefore, it is vital to be aware of the different types of programs and options available to you so that you are able to make an informed choice. A registered dietitian can design a safe and effective program for you to follow.

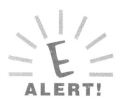

ALERT!

Women who have more than 15 to 20 pounds to lose, have health problems, or are taking medications on a regular basis should see their doctor before beginning any weight-loss program.

Once you reach your healthy goal weight, the key is to make it permanent and not begin a continuous cycle of yo-yo dieting (or losing and gaining weight). It is important to have the right motivation to maintain weight. Internal motivators such as health, a healthy pregnancy, increased energy, self-esteem, and feeling in control will increase the chances of lifelong success. The probability of long-term maintenance of goals is enhanced in those who exercise regularly, use social support to maintain their eating and exercise habits, interpret lapses positively as solvable problems, and view their eating and exercise regimens as permanent lifestyle habits rather then temporary measures.

Losing Weight Sensibly

The number of calories you consume and the number of calories you burn each day control your body weight. To lose weight, you need to consume fewer calories than you burn. The most successful way to do this is to become more physically active and moderately decrease the number of calories you eat. Most women, on average, need to consume about 1,200 to 1,400 calories daily, depending on factors such as age and activity level, to safely lose weight. Try to become physically active by walking or doing some other form of aerobic activity thirty minutes a day most days of the week.

Keep in mind that the type of calories you eat is also important. Those calories should come from the healthy foods that make up the Food Guide Pyramid (illustrated on page 3), such as fruits, vegetables, whole grains, fat-free or low-fat dairy products, lean meats, fish, poultry, and legumes. Watching your portion sizes carefully within each food group will help you keep you within a moderate calorie level. Keep in mind that a gradual weight loss increases your chances of keeping the weight off. Losing weight on your own does not need to be a difficult task. Follow some of these other guidelines to lose weight the smart way:

- Eat no more than 30 percent of your total calories from fat (about 40 grams of fat on a 1,200 calorie diet).
- Include at least five servings of fruit and vegetables in your diet each day as well as whole grains. Fiber can help you feel fuller.
- Choose fat-free and lower-fat products over those containing more fat. But don't forget that fat-free does not mean calorie-free!
- Plan your meals and snacks ahead of time—thinking ahead can save you calories.
- If you bolt your food, slow down! Eating slower can help you eat less.
- Examine your eating habits by keeping a written journal of what and when you eat.
- Expect temptation and plan some alternative strategies ahead of time.

- Weigh yourself once a week. Weighing yourself more frequently can be discouraging because weight fluctuates daily with changes in fluid balance.
- Eat breakfast as well as at least four to six small meals per day to help curb binge eating later in the day.

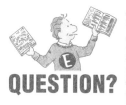

QUESTION?

I am overweight and trying to get pregnant. Is it okay to diet?
Strict dieting when planning to become pregnant is not recommended, especially if you leave out certain food groups, eat too few calories, or are on a ketone-promoting diet. Strict dieting can drastically affect the supply of nutrients that is vital for a healthy pregnancy and baby. Women who diet strictly in the years before becoming pregnant may be at higher risk for having low birth-weight babies. If you are concerned about your weight while trying to conceive, stick to a sensible eating plan along with regular exercise. A registered dietitian can help you to design a diet that is right for you.

Gaining Weight Sensibly

If you are under your healthy weight and need to add some pounds, you must do it in a healthy manner. Just because you need to gain weight doesn't mean you should eat whatever you want. You should still eat a healthy diet and just eat more of it. When choosing foods, choose healthy ones with concentrated calories. That way you don't need to increase the portion size as much. These foods can include peanut butter, dried fruits, avocados, nuts, and cheese. Try fortifying soups and casseroles with dry milk powder, or try supplements such as Carnation Instant Breakfast to add calories to your intake. Eat more frequently if your appetite is small and avoid drinking fluids close to mealtime so that you don't fill up too easily. A registered dietitian can help with weight gain as well as weight loss.

Existing Health Problems

If you are currently being treated for a chronic health problem such as diabetes, high blood pressure, thyroid disease, systemic lupus, seizure disorder, inflammatory bowel disease, asthma, heart problems, migraines, or any other condition, you should speak with your doctor before you try to conceive to understand how your health could affect your pregnancy. Your doctor may need to refer you to a specialist and/or change or eliminate certain medications to reduce any possible risk to the fetus. You may have to be much more vigilant about managing your condition and make sure your condition is well under control before you become pregnant.

In addition, you should ensure that all regular medical screening is up to date before you try to conceive. This may include annual pap smears, mammograms (for women over thirty-five), cholesterol screening, and diabetic screening. This should include your partner also. Making sure you are both healthy before you try to conceive can increase your chances of becoming pregnant.

Your Family History

Some conditions or diseases are genetic, recurring throughout some family histories. Examples include hemophilia (a blood disorder), sickle-cell anemia, cystic fibrosis, Tay-Sachs, thalassemia (or Cooley's anemia), celiac disease, Gaucher disease, Canavan disease, Niemann-Pick disease, and some birth defects. If you or your partner has a family history of a significant genetic disorder, and you suspect that either of you may be a carrier, then genetic testing may be advised. A carrier does not necessarily have the disorder but does carry a gene that could be passed on to the next generation. You should discuss your concerns with your doctor or health-care provider before you get pregnant.

Chapter 3

Eating for Two

Congratulations! Finally, you're pregnant! Now it is time to focus not just on yourself but on your baby, too. There is much to learn about how to properly nourish yourself and your growing baby. This chapter will help you eat your way through a healthy pregnancy. Please note that the intake requirements and recommended daily allowances described in this chapter are for women aged nineteen to fifty. Women outside this range may have slightly different requirements.

Am I Really Eating for Two?

Once you become pregnant, you may hear comments like, "Go ahead and eat, you are eating for two now." It is true that you need nutrients through the foods you choose for both you and the healthy development of your baby. Eating plenty of nutritionally dense foods—as opposed to junk that contains calories but very little nutrition—is the way to supply your baby with all the nutrition he needs. On the other hand, you don't need to eat enough calories for two. In fact, eating too much can cause unnecessary weight gain. At the same time, eating too little may keep your baby from receiving all of the nutrition he needs. The key is to keep a healthy balance.

Calorie needs increase slightly during pregnancy to help support a woman's maternal body changes and the baby's proper growth and development. It is true that your body requires more calories during pregnancy, but "more" here means only a moderate amount. After the first trimester, you need about 300 calories per day above your maintenance level. That adds up to about 85,000 calories over the nine months that you are pregnant. Calorie needs will be more if you are carrying more than one baby. Your extra daily calorie needs will jump to 500 calories if you breastfeed following pregnancy. It does not take much to consume an extra 300 calories. The key is to choose nutrient-rich foods that contain plenty of lean protein, complex carbohydrates, fiber, vitamins, and minerals for your extra calories. An extra 300 calories can translate to any of the following:

- A 6-ounce baked potato, with skin, topped with 2 ounces of low-fat cheese, ½ cup of broccoli, and ¼ cup of salsa
- ½ cup tuna salad, half a piece of pita bread, lettuce, tomato, with 1 tablespoon low-fat mayo
- 8 ounces skim milk or 8 oz. low-fat yogurt, a banana, ¼ cup low-fat granola

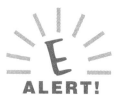

ALERT!

Skipping meals during pregnancy can have serious effects on the proper development of the baby. Skipping meals will force the baby to go too long without proper nourishment, and it can sabotage your efforts to consume enough healthy calories each day.

Determining Your Calorie Needs

There are many different methods for estimating caloric needs. It is important to remember that these methods result only in estimates; still, you can get a general idea of the number of calories your body needs. Everyone's caloric needs differ, depending on factors such as age, gender, size, body composition, basal metabolic rate, and physical activity.

Basal metabolic rate (BMR) is the number of calories your body would burn if you were at rest all day. By figuring your basal metabolic rate, you know the minimum number of calories you must consume to maintain your weight. On average, a moderately active woman needs between 1,800 and 2,200 calories per day. A pregnant woman needs about 2,500 calories after the first trimester. However, because you don't spend every day lying in bed, you have additional calorie needs on top of your basal rate. The next section describes how to determine the number of calories you should ingest every day.

You Do the Math

Use this simple equation to figure your basic calorie needs:

1. First, figure your basal metabolic rate to get the minimum number of calories your body needs to maintain a healthy weight. To do this, multiply your healthy weight (in pounds) by 10. For instance, a woman whose healthy weight is 165 pounds would have a basal metabolic rate of 1,650—in other words, this woman needs to take in a minimum of 1,650 calories to maintain her body weight. (If you are overweight, use the average weight within the range given on the Healthy Weight Chart provided in Chapter 2. Using your actual weight if you are overweight may overestimate your calorie needs.)
2. Figure how many additional calories you need to sustain your level of physical activity. To do this, choose the activity level from the following list that best describes you and take the appropriate percentage of your basal metabolic rate.
   - **Sedentary**—You mainly engage in low-intensity activities throughout your day, such as sitting, driving a car, lying down, sleeping,

standing, typing, or reading. Take 20 percent of your basal metabolic rate (multiply by 0.2).

- **Light activity**—Your day includes light exercise, such as walking, but for no more than two hours of your day. Take 30 percent of your basal metabolic rate (multiply by 0.3).
- **Moderate activity**—You engage in moderate exercise throughout the day, such as heavy housework, gardening, dancing, with very little sitting. Take 40 percent of your basal metabolic rate (multiply by 0.4).
- **High activity**—You engage in active physical sports or have a labor-intensive job, such as construction work, on a daily basis. Take 50 percent of your basal metabolic rate (multiply by 0.5).

3. Figure out how many additional calories you need to sustain your body's digestion and absorption of nutrients. To do this, add your results from steps 1 and 2, then take 10 percent of the total (multiply by 0.1).

4. To find your total calorie needs, add your basal metabolic rate from step 1, the calories to sustain your level of physical activity from step 2, and the number of calories needed for digestion from step 3. Take the example of the 165-pound woman from step 1, with the basal metabolic rate of 1,650. She is moderately active, which means she needs an additional 660 calories to sustain her activity level. She needs 231 calories to fuel her body's digestion and food absorption processes ($1,650 + 660 \times 0.1 = 231$). Adding those values gives us a total of 2,541, which is the total number of calories a moderately active 165-pound woman should ingest to maintain her weight.

5. To account for the additional calories you need to sustain your body weight during pregnancy, add 300 to the total from step 4. This final value represents your estimated basic calorie needs.

A Little Extra Help

Doing the math will only give you an estimate of your calorie needs. Some women have special needs. If you are having problems figuring out your calorie needs, or if you are not sure what to eat to get those extra calories in, don't hesitate to contact a registered dietitian to help you out. Some women may need a little extra nutritional help to ensure they are getting everything that they need. It is recommended that you seek extra help if you are younger than seventeen or older than thirty-five, pregnant with more than one baby, underweight or overweight prior to becoming pregnant, a strict vegetarian, lactose intolerant, gaining too much or too little during pregnancy, having trouble eating due to nausea and/or vomiting, on a special diet due to allergies, diabetes, or gastrointestinal or digestive disorder, or if you have suffered with eating disorders. Don't go it alone if you are not sure what to do. Nutrition and calorie intake is vital to a healthy baby and a healthy pregnancy. Never hesitate to ask for help!

The Pregnancy Food Guide Pyramid

Eating a variety of foods from all of the food groups is the best way to ensure you are getting the calories and nutrients you need. The USDA's Food Guide Pyramid is a good guideline for pregnant women; it ensures you consume the following minimum number of servings in each food group (about 2,500 calories):

- 9 servings from the bread, cereal, rice, and pasta group. Examples of a single serving from this group include a slice of whole-wheat bread, ½ cup cooked cereal, half a bagel, or ½ cup of pasta. Be sure to include whole-grain and whole-wheat starches as well as other starches higher in fiber.
- 4 servings from the vegetable group. Examples of a single serving from this group include 1 cup of raw leafy vegetables, ½ cup of other vegetables, raw or cooked, or ¾ cup vegetable juice. Choose a variety of vegetables—the darker the color, the more nutrients a vegetable has.
- 3 servings from the fruit group. Examples of a single serving from this group include a medium apple, a small banana, a small orange, ½ cup chopped fruit, or ¾ cup fruit juice. Choose a variety of fruits daily, as raw fruits are higher in fiber than juices.
- 3–4 servings from the milk, yogurt, and cheese group. Examples of a single serving from this group include 1 cup of milk or yogurt, 1.5 ounces natural cheese, or 2 ounces processed cheese. Use fat-free or low-fat milk, nonfat or low-fat yogurt, and low-fat cheese.

- 6–7 ounces (2–3 servings) from the meat, poultry, fish, dry beans, eggs, and nuts group. Examples of a single serving from this group include 3 ounces poultry, fish, or lean meat; 1 ounce meat = ½ cup cooked dried beans, a whole egg, ½ cup tofu, ⅓ cup nuts, or 2 tablespoons peanut butter. Choose lean meats and trim fat from meat before cooking. With poultry, remove skin. Include cooked dry beans often as the main dish in meals.

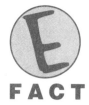

FACT

A common pitfall to the healthy diet is skipping breakfast. When you skip breakfast, you are forcing your body to go ten to twelve hours without food—and going that long without nourishing your baby. When you are famished, it is easy to choose the wrong foods and eat too much of them, so skipping breakfast may cause you to eat more calories than you intended.

Carving Up the Calories

The calories in all the healthy foods that make up the USDA Food Guide Pyramid are made up of three basic nutrients: carbohydrates, protein, and fat. These three nutrients are known as the macronutrients because we need them in larger amounts. Even though each macronutrient has a particular function in the body, they work together in partnership for good health and for a healthy pregnancy. During pregnancy, the required amounts of some of these nutrients change only slightly.

Count on Carbohydrates

You can count on carbohydrates to be your body's main source of energy, especially for the brain and nervous system. Carbohydrates quickly and efficiently convert to energy for mom and baby. Carbohydrates are found in fruits, vegetables, dairy products, starches, and foods in the meat group such as beans and soy products. The only foods in which they are not found are meat, poultry, and fish. Fiber is also considered a carbohydrate and is important to health. However, fiber is not considered a nutrient because most of it is not digested or absorbed into the body.

Comprehending Carbs

Carbohydrates are classified into two different categories: simple carbohydrates, or sugars, and complex carbohydrates, or starches. Sugars are carbohydrates in their simplest form. Refined sugars are found in foods such as table sugar, honey, jams, candy, syrup, and soft drinks. Refined sugars provide calories, but they lack nutrients like vitamins and minerals, and fiber. Some simple sugars, such as those that occur naturally, are found in more nutritious foods, such as the fructose found in fruit or the lactose that is part of dairy products. Complex carbohydrates are basically formed of many simple sugars linked together. They are found in foods such as grains, pasta, rice, vegetables, breads, legumes, nuts, and seeds. Complex carbohydrates are much more nutrient-rich than simple sugars.

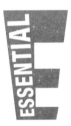

Before complex or simple carbohydrates can be used as energy, they must be broken down into glucose, or blood sugar. Glucose is carried through your bloodstream to your body's cells, where it is converted to energy. Since simple carbohydrates or sugars are already in their simplest form, they go straight into the bloodstream. Complex carbohydrates must be broken down into glucose. Some glucose is used as energy, and some is stored. The hormone insulin helps to regulate your blood sugar.

How Many Carbs?

On average, women should get approximately 45 to 65 percent of their calories from carbohydrates. Since pregnancy increases calorie needs, more calories must be ingested from carbohydrates. The key is to increase your calories by eating more complex carbohydrates and not more sugar. Take in more complex carbohydrates by eating more fruits and vegetables, whole grains, rice, breads, and cereals. Try adding more beans, lentils, and peas to your daily meals.

To figure how many grams of carbohydrates you need, follow these steps:

1. Calculate your estimated calorie need, as described on page 33.
2. Multiply your total by .45 (at the low end of recommended carb intake) to up to .65 (at the high end). The result is the number of calories you should get from carbohydrates.
3. Calculate the number of grams of carbohydrates you need to eat as follows. Take the number of carbohydrate calories (from step 2) and divide by 4. Carbohydrates contain 4 calories per gram, so the result of this step is the total grams of carbohydrates you should eat daily.

Following the Food Guide Pyramid and eating the suggested number of servings from each food group during pregnancy will ensure you are consuming the amount of carbohydrates your body needs for a healthy pregnancy and a healthy baby. Even though carbohydrates are extremely important, they need to be balanced with the other two macronutrients: protein and fat.

Powerful Protein

Protein is a powerful macronutrient. During pregnancy, protein provides the material needed for the physical growth and cellular development of the growing baby. Protein is also needed to build the mother's placenta, amniotic tissue, and other maternal tissues. A woman's blood volume increases by almost 50 percent during pregnancy, and additional protein is needed to produce those new blood cells.

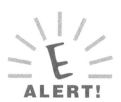

ALERT!

A low protein intake during pregnancy can increase the risk of having a low birth-weight baby. These babies are more prone to health problems and learning disabilities later in life.

During your pregnancy, you need slightly more protein than you did before, and during breastfeeding your needs will continue to increase. The body does not store protein, so you must consume a continuous supply. You need about 10 extra grams of protein from your extra daily calories, or 60 grams of protein daily, compared with the 50 grams a non-pregnant woman requires. Women expecting multiple babies may need more. Here are some examples of where you might find an extra 10 grams of protein:

- In a 1.5-ounce serving of lean meat
- In about 10 ounces of fat-free milk
- In 1.5 ounces of canned tuna in water

Most women do not have a problem meeting their protein requirements. Eating plenty of lean meat, fish, eggs, legumes, and dried beans as well as increasing your dairy servings will ensure you meet your protein needs. If you are a vegetarian and consume plenty of legumes, grain products, vegetables, fruits, and soy foods, you should not have a problem consuming the recommended amount of protein.

Face the Fat

Fat is an important nutrient that sometimes gets a bad rap. Its major functions in the body include providing an energy source, aiding in the absorption and transport of the fat-soluble vitamins A, D, E, and K, cushioning organs, and regulating body temperature. All women, pregnant or not, should get 20 to 35 percent of their calories from fat. Fat can be dangerous to health if consumed in excess or if the wrong kinds of fat are eaten. It is important to include fat in your daily diet but in moderation. Fat is a very concentrated source of calories. A gram of fat has 9 calories, twice as many as a gram of carbohydrates or protein (both of which contain 4 calories per gram). A small amount of fat can go a long way!

How Many Fats Are There?

There are different types of triglycerides, or dietary fats. Some of these fats are more harmful than others. The major kinds of fats in the foods we eat are saturated, polyunsaturated, monounsaturated, and trans-fatty acids or hydrogenated fats. The unsaturated fats (polyunsaturated and monounsaturated) are referred to as the "healthy" fats. These fats can help to lower cholesterol levels, and they also have heart-protective factors. Most of the fat in your diet should be unsaturated.

Sources of monounsaturated fats include certain plant-based oils, such as olive, canola, and peanut. Avocados are also good sources of monounsaturated fats. Sources of polyunsaturated fats include certain other plant-based oils such as corn, cottonseed, safflower, sunflower, sesame, and soybean. Nuts and seeds are also good sources. This group also includes the omega-3 fatty acids found in some fish. There are two polyunsaturated essential fatty acids that your body does not make and you must get from the food you consume. These two fatty acids are linoleic acid (or omega-6) and linolenic acid (or omega-3).

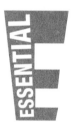

Eating a totally fat-free diet is not part of a healthy eating style. Fat is an essential nutrient, and some fats—such as omega-3 fatty acids—are necessary for certain parts of a baby's development. A totally fat-free diet may also fail to provide sufficient calories.

Saturated fats and trans-fatty acids tend to increase blood cholesterol levels, which can lead to health problems such as heart disease and stroke. The major sources of saturated fat are animal foods such as meat, poultry, and whole-milk dairy products. However, some plant sources also provide saturated fat, including palm, palm kernel, and coconut oils. Food that contains trans-fats includes some margarines, cookies, crackers, and other commercial baked goods made with partially hydrogenated vegetable oils, as well as French fries, donuts, and other commercial fried foods.

Slash the Fat

Fat is definitely a needed nutrient in a healthy diet. The problem is that most Americans consume too much and the wrong kinds. Don't cut fat completely out of your diet, but it is important to cut back and to choose the right types. This means lowering your intake of dietary cholesterol and saturated fat. You should also lower your blood cholesterol or maintain it at safe levels as a way of decreasing your risk for heart disease. You can cut the fat and cholesterol from your meals without losing any flavor. For example, try using egg whites or egg substitute in place of whole eggs. Choose leaner meats, cook with skinless poultry and fish, or occasionally opt for a vegetarian meal with beans or soy products as your main protein source. Read the nutrition facts panel to keep an eye on your daily intake of total fat, saturated fat, and cholesterol.

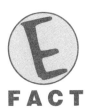

FACT

Cholesterol is not the same as fat. Cholesterol is a fat-like substance, but it has a different structure and different functions in the body than fat does. Because cholesterol provides no energy to the body, it has no calories.

Apply the Brakes on Sugar

How bad is sugar? In moderation, it can be part of a healthy diet. Sugar belongs to the carbohydrate group, which also includes starches and fibers. Natural sugars are found in fruit (in the form of fructose) and milk (as lactose). Sugar becomes a dietary culprit when it is added to other foods (usually processed items). Major sources of added sugar are those found in soft drinks, candy, pastries, cookies, ice cream, and other sweets. Although the body does not know the difference between sugar and complex carbohydrates, most sugars are referred to as "empty calories" because they provide calories but very little or no nutritional value. Satisfy your sweet tooth, but do it in moderation.

How Much Is Too Much?

The typical American diet is packed with too much sugar, and nutrition experts agree that Americans need to cut back. The idea behind a healthy pregnancy diet is to eat foods that really count toward your nutritional intake. Eating too many sugary foods means lots of extra calories and very little nutrition. Eating too many of these foods also tends to bump out the more nutritious foods that you should be choosing. Foods with lots of added sugar should only be occasional treats, not regular snacks.

Though there is no established recommended daily allowance (RDA) for sugar, you should concentrate of getting the bulk of your carbohydrates from complex sources—such as breads, rice, and pasta—and most of your simple carbohydrates from fruits and dairy products, which also contain vitamins, minerals, and fiber.

Sweet, Sweet Food Labels

The FDA requires sugar content to be included on all nutrition facts panels. The panel lists total carbohydrates and sugar in terms of grams per serving. Sugar is part of the total carbohydrate amount that is listed. If you purchase a food with added sugar, make sure it also provides plenty of nutrients such as vitamins and minerals, and fiber.

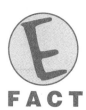

FACT

When checking the ingredient labels on packaged food, you will find all types of sweeteners listed. The suffix "-ose" (fructose, sucrose, lactose) indicates that an ingredient is a form of sugar. Look for these other ingredients that indicate added sugar: brown sugar, corn sweetener, corn syrup, fruit juice concentrate, high-fructose corn syrup, honey, invert sugar, lactose, molasses, and raw sugar.

If you see a nutritional claim with the word "sugar" on the front of a packaged label, it is important to understand what that claim means.

What It Says	What It Means
Calorie-free	Less than 5 calories
Sugar-free	Less than 0.5 grams sugar per serving
Reduced sugar or less sugar	At least 25% less* sugar or sugars per serving
No added sugars, without added sugars, no sugar	No sugars added during processing or packing, including ingredients that contain sugar such as juice or dry fruit

*As compared with a standard serving size of the traditional food.

Use these guidelines to help you choose foods wisely to ensure you're getting the nutrition you need to help grow a healthy baby.

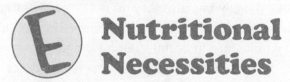

Chapter 4

Nutritional Necessities

A healthy pregnancy diet needs a balance of all components. That includes important macronutrients, micronutrients (including vitamins and minerals), as well as overlooked nutrients such as water, and fiber. It is important to recognize whether you are getting what you need for a healthy pregnancy and to make necessary changes in your daily diet if you are not.

Priceless Vitamins

Vitamins are known as micronutrients because we need them in much smaller amounts than carbohydrates, proteins, and fats. Even though you need them in smaller amounts, that does not make them any less important. Vitamins are involved in all kinds of functions throughout the body. They don't supply energy directly because they do not provide any calories to the body, but vitamins do regulate many of the processes that produce energy. Although all vitamins are important during pregnancy—and you should concentrate on getting enough of all of them—some deserve special attention. Vitamins fall into two categories: water-soluble and fat-soluble vitamins.

Fat-Soluble Vitamins

The fat-soluble vitamins include vitamins A, D, E, and K. Fat-soluble vitamins dissolve in fat, and they travel throughout the body by attaching to body chemicals made with fat. These vitamins can be stored in the body, so it can be harmful to consume more than you need over a long period of time.

Vitamin A

Vitamin A promotes the growth and the health of cells and tissues for both the mother and the baby. In the form of beta-carotene, vitamin A also acts as a powerful antioxidant. We have already discussed the dangers of too much vitamin A and its relationship to birth defects. Beta-carotene, which forms vitamin A, does not pose any danger to expectant mothers. Your body converts beta-carotene to vitamin A only when the body needs it. The recommended daily allowance (RDA) of vitamin A is measured in micrograms (mcg). In supplements and on nutrition facts panels, it is measured in international units (IU). The need for vitamin A increases only slightly during pregnancy, from 700 to 770 mcg (for women nineteen to fifty years of age).

Vitamin D

Another important fat-soluble vitamin during pregnancy is vitamin D. This vitamin aids in calcium balance and helps your body absorb sufficient calcium for you and your baby. Vitamin D is known as the "sunshine vitamin" because the body can make vitamin D after sunlight hits the skin. It is important to get enough vitamin D throughout your life as a way of helping to avoid osteoporosis (or brittle bone disease). Since vitamin D is stored in the body, too much can be toxic. Excess amounts usually come from supplements and not food or too much sunlight. During pregnancy, women should get 5 mcg per day.

Water-Soluble Vitamins

The water-soluble vitamin group consists of the B-complex vitamins and vitamin C. Water-soluble vitamins dissolve in water and are then carried in your bloodstream. Most are not stored in the body in any significant amounts. What your body does not use is excreted through the urine. Since they are not stored in the body, water-soluble vitamins pose less of a risk for toxicity (though moderation is still the best approach). This also means that you need a regular supply from your diet.

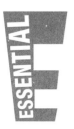

The B-complex vitamins are a family of vitamins that all work together and have similar functions in health. They include vitamin B_1 (thiamin), vitamin B_2 (riboflavin), niacin, vitamin B_6, folate, vitamin B_{12}, biotin, and pantothenic acid. Most B vitamins help the body to indirectly produce energy within its cells.

Folic Acid

Folic acid is a B vitamin whose main role is to maintain the cell's genetic code or DNA (the cell's master plan for cell reproduction). It also works with vitamin B_{12} to form hemoglobin in red blood cells. Folic acid has gained much attention for its role in reducing the risk for neural tube birth defects, such as spina bifida, in newborn babies. Other risks of folic acid deficiencies include anemia, impaired growth, and abnormal digestive function. It is vital that pregnant women or women of childbearing years consume enough folic acid through food and supplements, especially during the first trimester.

Before pregnancy a woman's need for folic acid is 400 mcg per day. During pregnancy, that amount jumps to 600 mcg per day. Recent studies show that to decrease the risk of birth defects, women planning a pregnancy should increase their daily intake of folic acid to 800 to 1,000 mcg. Most prenatal vitamins contain 800 to 1,000 mcg to ensure that women fully absorb the amount they need during pregnancy to help decrease the risk of birth defects. Taking too much folic acid through supplements can mask a vitamin B_{12} deficiency and could interfere with some medications. However, some women may need more folic acid with certain medications.

Other B Vitamins

Vitamin B_6 is necessary in helping your body make nonessential amino acids (the building blocks of protein). These nonessential amino acids are used to make necessary body cells. Vitamin B_6 also helps to turn the amino acid tryptophan into niacin and serotonin (a messenger in the brain). In addition to those functions, this vitamin helps produce insulin, hemoglobin, and antibodies that help fight infection. Requirements are increased slightly in pregnancy due to the needs of the baby. The recommended level during pregnancy is 1.9 mg.

Requirements are also increased for vitamin B_{12} during pregnancy to help with the formation of red blood cells. The increase is slight, from 2.4 mcg before pregnancy to 2.6 mcg during pregnancy. This vitamin is found mostly in foods of animal origin, so vegetarians need a reliable source of vitamin B_{12}, such as fortified breakfast cereal or supplements.

Vitamin C

Vitamin C produces collagen, a connective tissue that holds muscles, bones, and other tissues together. In addition it helps with a variety of other functions, including forming and repairing red blood cells, bones, and other tissue; protecting you from bruising by keeping capillary walls and blood vessels firm; keeping your gums healthy; healing cuts and wounds; and keeping your immune system strong and healthy. Vitamin C also helps your body absorb iron from plant sources, which is not as easily absorbed as iron from animals. Vitamin C is one of the very powerful antioxidants that attacks free radicals (unstable molecules with a missing electron formed when the body's cells burn oxygen) in the body's fluids. These free radicals can damage the body's cells, tissues, and even DNA (your body's master plan for reproducing cells).

With pregnancy, a woman's need for vitamin C increases slightly, from 75 mg to 85 mg (for women nineteen to fifty years). Because vitamin C is so readily available in numerous food sources, it is not difficult to get the extra you need.

Don't Miss Your Minerals

Minerals are also known as micronutrients. As with vitamins, your good health and your healthy pregnancy require an optimal supply. Minerals do not supply energy to the body directly, because they do not contain calories, but they do fulfill many vital functions. Minerals are part of a baby's bones and teeth. Along with protein and certain vitamins, minerals help to produce blood cells and other body tissues. Minerals aid in numerous body functions that support a normal pregnancy.

Minerals are categorized as either major minerals or trace minerals. Though they are all important, trace minerals are needed in smaller amounts than major minerals. Minerals are absorbed into your intestines and then are transported and stored in your body in various ways. Some minerals pass directly into your bloodstream. They are then transported to the cells, and the excess passes out of the body through the urine. Again, the rule of moderation is the best policy. Although all minerals are important during pregnancy and you should concentrate on getting enough of all of them, some deserve special attention.

Calcium

We already know how vital calcium is to strong bones and teeth. We also know that if your growing baby can't get what she needs, the fetal development process will rob your calcium stores. You need enough calcium to protect your stores and for the development of the baby's bones. Consuming enough calcium during pregnancy may also reduce your chances of developing high blood pressure and toxemia. Calcium requirements do not change throughout pregnancy, but many women still don't consume enough. Regardless of whether you are pregnant, you should consume at least 1,000 mg per day (for women aged nineteen to fifty years). If you do not consume enough calcium-containing foods, such as dairy products, speak to your doctor about calcium supplements. Keep in mind that the upper limit for calcium is 2,500 mg per day.

Iron

As your blood volume increases during the time you are pregnant, your iron needs increase as well. Iron is essential for making hemoglobin, the component of blood that carries oxygen throughout the body and to the baby. Foods rich in vitamin C can help iron be absorbed into the blood. Many women start their pregnancies with less than optimal stores of iron, which can increase their risk of becoming anemic. Women who have iron deficiency anemia may be prescribed a higher dose of iron supplements. You should never increase your iron intake, especially through supplements, without first speaking with your doctor.

Zinc

Almost every cell in the body contains zinc, which is also part of over seventy different types of enzymes. Zinc is known as the second most abundant trace mineral in the human body. Your requirement for this mineral increases slightly during pregnancy from 8 to 11 mg (for women nineteen to fifty years). Zinc is needed for cell growth and brain development. Too much iron from supplements can inhibit the absorption of zinc.

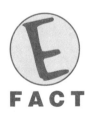

FACT

Women who are having multiple babies have slightly higher recommended intakes for some vitamins and minerals. Your doctor can advise you as to your recommended nutritional intake.

Don't Rule Out Sodium

Although sodium sometimes gets bad press, it is still a mineral that is essential to life and to good health—and that also means during pregnancy. Sodium has many important functions in the body, such as controlling the flow of fluids in and out of each cell, regulating blood pressure, transmitting nerve impulses, and helping your muscles relax (including the heart, which is a muscle.) Sodium, chloride, and potassium are known as electrolytes, compounds that transmit electrical currents through the body. As a result of these currents, nerve impulses can also be transmitted.

Recommended Amounts

The terms "salt" and "sodium" are often used interchangeably, yet they are two different things. Sodium is an element of table salt, which is technically known as "sodium chloride." How much sodium is in table salt? A single teaspoon of salt contains 2,000 mg of sodium. Generally, articles and guidelines that warn of the dangers of eating too much salt are concerned with sodium only.

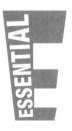

Fluid retention, or edema, is very normal during pregnancy and is not always the result of eating too much sodium. Instead, this condition is usually the result of increased estrogen production and a greater blood volume. Do not decrease your sodium intake to relieve edema. Restricting sodium too much can disrupt the body's fluid balance. Extra fluids, especially water, can help relieve some edema. If you are experiencing excessive edema, see your doctor before making any dietary changes.

Although pregnant women should not decrease their sodium intake, excessive intake is not recommended either. During pregnancy, your body's need for sodium increases. Most women get plenty of sodium in their regular diets, and it is almost never necessary to arrange for extra sodium. In fact, the typical American consumes 4,000 to 8,000 mg per day, well above daily recommended levels. The moderate goal for adults, including pregnant and breastfeeding women, is approximately 2,400 mg of sodium per day.

In healthy people, the kidneys help regulate the sodium level in the body. Sodium levels usually don't become too high because most excess sodium is excreted from the body in urine and through perspiration. For example, when you eat foods that are high in salt, you probably urinate more frequently because the body is trying to rid itself of the extra sodium. Even though your sodium intake may vary from day to day, your body is very efficient at maintaining a proper balance.

Moderate Your Sodium Intake

While sodium is a very important mineral during pregnancy, be careful not to overdo it. For many people, consuming sodium in moderation means making some dietary and lifestyle changes. A strong preference for salty foods is easily acquired and usually starts at a young age. It is all in what your taste buds get used to. To help moderate the amount of sodium in your diet, begin to gradually decrease your salt intake, especially if you are accustomed to salty tastes. Eat plenty of fresh or frozen fruits and vegetables as well as fresh foods as opposed to processed, canned, or prepared foods. If you eat frozen convenience foods often, look for products that have less than 800 mg sodium per serving. Choose lower sodium foods by paying attention to the nutrition facts panel on all packaged foods. Keep in mind that condiments such as ketchup, soy sauce, teriyaki sauce, mustard, pickles, and olives can be high in sodium, so go easy on these.

Fill Up on Fluids

Water is a nutrient that is just as important as macronutrients and micronutrients. Water acts as your body's transportation system to carry nutrients to your body cells as well as your baby's. Water helps to regulate body temperature through perspiration and by transporting oxygen through the body, carrying waste products away from the body cells, cushioning joints, and protecting body organs. Proper hydration before, during, and after is a vital component of a healthy pregnancy.

How Much to Drink

Pregnant women need extra fluid to support their increased blood volume and for amniotic fluid. Because the body has no provision to store water, the amount of water you lose each day must be continually replaced to maintain proper hydration. During both pregnancy and breastfeeding, women should aim to drink eight to twelve 8-ounce glasses of water per day. This may increase if you are perspiring in hot weather, when exercising, or if you have any type of fever, diarrhea, or vomiting. Inadequate water intake can lead to problems like fatigue, muscle weakness, and headaches, just to name a few. For the fetus, dehydration can affect adequate nutrient transport, induce poor waste removal, create too warm an environment, and decrease cushioning. These can all affect fetal growth and development. Being properly hydrated can help to reduce swelling and bothersome constipation. Staying properly hydrated can help you to feel more energized, give you an improved sense of well being, provide greater endurance and stamina during physical activity, and improve your digestion and elimination.

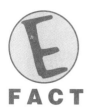

FACT

Water contributes close to 55 to 65 percent of an adult's body weight, and during pregnancy your body's water needs expand substantially. Water is present in every part of your body: 83 percent of blood, 73 percent of muscle, 25 percent of body fat, and even 22 percent of bones are made up of water.

The best and easiest way to get your fluids is simply by drinking water. Other fluids that can contribute to your daily intake include fat-free or low-fat milk, club soda, bottled water, vegetable juice, seltzer, and fruit juice. Be careful of drinking too many beverages, such as juice, that are healthy but also pack in a lot of calories. Stay clear of alcohol and most herbal teas, and limit coffee, tea, soft drinks, diet soft drinks, and other caffeinated beverages. If you feel thirsty, your body is telling you that it is already becoming dehydrated, so drink up.

Drink, Drank, Drunk

Like everything else, drinking water should be part of your healthy life-style—you should make it a habit. Make a commitment today to start drinking water on a regular basis. You should be in the habit before you even become pregnant. You should start out with a moderate goal and work your way up. It may help to start a water diary on a calendar to keep track of your current intake and your progress. If you need help increasing your water intake, follow some of these helpful tips:

- At work or at home, take water breaks instead of coffee breaks.
- Keep a bottle of water at your desk, on your counter at home, or in your car when traveling so you have it available to sip throughout the day.
- Get in the habit of drinking a glass of water before and with meals and snacks. Besides helping you to stay hydrated, it can help take the edge off of your appetite.
- Use a straw to drink your water. Believe it or not, using a straw can help you drink faster and make a glass of water seem a little more manageable.
- Drink water instead of snacking while watching television or reading a book.
- Keep a two-quart container of water in the refrigerator, and make it your goal to drink it all by the end of the day. This also gives you a constant supply of good, cold water.

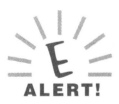

ALERT!

It is normal to get thirsty once in awhile, but if you are excessively thirsty and find yourself drinking large amounts of water, this could be a sign of a medical condition such as diabetes. If you feel you are drinking because of severe thirst, as opposed to a healthy habit, speak to your doctor.

Fabulous Fiber

Fiber is exclusively found in plant foods; it is the part of the plant that our bodies cannot digest. Fiber, also called dietary fiber, is categorized as a complex carbohydrate, but because it cannot be digested or absorbed into your bloodstream, it is not considered a nutrient. There are two types of fiber: soluble and insoluble. Each type has a different beneficial health function in the body. It is important to eat a variety of fiber-rich foods every day that will provide you with the health benefits of both soluble and insoluble fiber.

Soluble Fibers

Soluble fibers naturally found in plants include gums, mucilages, psyllium, and pectins. Foods that contain these fibers include peas, beans, oats, barley, and some fruits (especially apples with skin, oranges, prunes, strawberries, and bananas) and some vegetables (especially carrots, broccoli, and cauliflower). Soluble fiber binds to fatty substances and promotes their excretion, which in turn seems to help lower blood cholesterol levels.

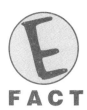

FACT

According to the American Heart Association, soluble fibers, when part of your everyday low-fat and low-cholesterol diet, can aid in slowing the absorption of sugar into the bloodstream, which in turn can help to control your blood sugar levels.

Insoluble Fibers

Insoluble fiber is known as "roughage." The insoluble fibers give plants their structure. Insoluble fibers naturally found in plants include cellulose, hemicellulose, and lignin. Foods that contain these fibers include whole-wheat or whole-grain products, wheat bran, corn bran, some fruits (especially the skin), and many vegetables including cauliflower, green beans, potatoes with skin, and broccoli. Insoluble fibers do not dissolve in water, but they hold on to water as they move waste through your intestinal tract. By holding on to water, they add bulk and softness to the stool and therefore promote regularity and help prevent constipation. Insoluble fibers also help accelerate intestinal transit time, which means they decrease the amount of time that waste stays in the colon. This cuts the time that potentially harmful waste food substances can linger in the intestines.

Fabulous Fiber Benefits

Fiber may not bring the word "fabulous" to your mind, but maybe it should. Basically, fiber comes in and goes out of the body. However, it does some pretty amazing things on its travels. Fiber helps to promote good health in many ways. Studies show that a diet rich in fiber as part of a varied, balanced, and low-fat eating pattern may help to prevent some chronic diseases. No matter how good your present health is, you can certainly benefit from adding more fiber to your diet. Fiber not only promotes health but also may help to reduce the risk for digestive problems, heart disease, some types of cancer, and diabetes. A fiber-rich diet can also help to promote weight management.

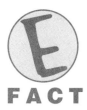

FACT

There is such a thing as too much of a good thing. Eating more than 50 or 60 grams of fiber per day may cause a decrease in the amount of vitamins and minerals, such as zinc, iron, magnesium and calcium, that your body absorbs. Large amounts of fiber can also cause gas, diarrhea, and bloating.

How Much Fiber?

A diet rich in fiber is important at all times, but it can be especially helpful during pregnancy. A fiber-rich diet can help to prevent constipation, which plagues many pregnant women. The average American only eats about 12 to 17 grams of fiber daily, which is well below the recommended levels, so make sure you make the necessary changes to your diet to boost your fiber! Adults under the age of fifty should get 25 grams a day; adults over fifty should get 21 grams. When boosting your fiber intake, it is important to increase your intake gradually and to make sure you are drinking plenty of fluids.

Getting Your Fill of Fiber

Adding fiber to your diet may be easier than you think. Just looking at the fiber content on the nutrition facts panel on packaged foods can help you be aware of what you need to do to increase your fiber intake. Choose foods that are good sources of fiber and have at least 2.5 grams or more of fiber per serving. Make simple switches by substituting higher-fiber foods, such as whole-grain breads, brown rice, whole-wheat pasta, fruits, and vegetables for lower-fiber foods such as white bread, white rice, candy, and chips. Eat more raw vegetables and fresh fruits, and include the skins when appropriate. Lightly steam these foods, which can preserve a lot of the fiber content. Plan your meals to include high-fiber foods such as fruits, vegetables, legumes, or whole-grain starches. Simply adding extra vegetables to your favorite sandwiches, soups, and casseroles can make a world of difference.

What better way to start your day than with a high-fiber breakfast cereal such as bran cereal or oatmeal? Look for cereals that contain at least 3 to 5 grams or more of fiber per serving. Add some fresh fruit to the top of your cereal for an extra fiber boost. Since both soluble and insoluble fibers are important for good health, eat a variety of high-fiber foods to ensure you get a mix of both types of fiber. Make good use of your snacks by choosing those that will increase your fiber intake. Nibble on dried fruits, popcorn, fresh fruit, raw vegetables, whole-wheat bagels, or whole-wheat crackers. Try something different and add legumes, or dried beans, to your diet at least two to three times per week. You can add them to salads, soups, casseroles, or spaghetti sauce.

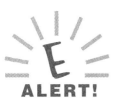

ALERT!

Don't rely on juice for daily servings of fruit. Whole fruits contain more fiber than juice because much of the fiber is found in the skin and pulp, which is removed when the juice is made.

Fiber-Rich Foods

There are a variety of foods that contain fiber. Try a variety and add fiber-rich foods to every meal.

Food	Serving Size	Fiber (grams)
FRUIT		
Apple with skin	1 medium	3
Banana	1 medium	2
Blueberries	½ cup	2
Figs, dried	2	4
Orange	1 medium	3
Orange juice	¾ cup	less than 1
Pear with skin	1 medium	4
Strawberries	1 cup	4
VEGETABLES		
Broccoli, cooked	½ cup	2
Brussels sprouts, cooked	½ cup	3
Carrots, raw	1 medium	2
Potato, baked with skin	1 medium	4
Spinach, cooked	½ cup	2
Tomato, raw	1 medium	2
NUTS/BEANS		
Beans/Lentils, cooked		
Baked beans	½ cup	3
Kidney beans	½ cup	3
Lentils	½ cup	4
Navy beans	½ cup	4
Peanut butter, chunky	2 T	1.5
White beans	½ cup	4.5

Food	Serving Size	Fiber (grams)
BREADS AND GRAINS		
Brown rice, cooked	½ cup	2
Pumpernickel bread	1 slice	3
Wheat bran	1 tablespoon	2
Whole-wheat bread	1 slice	2
CEREALS		
100% bran	1/3 cup	8
Bran flakes	¾ cup	5
Oatmeal, cooked	¾ cup	3
Raisin bran	¾ cup	5
SNACK FOODS		
Peanuts, dry-roasted	¼ cup	3
Popcorn, air-popped	1 cup	1
Sunflower seeds	¼ cup	2

Fiber Supplements

Many fiber supplements contain only small amounts of fiber compared with the amounts that are found in foods. With supplements that contain more fiber, it is easy to overdo your fiber intake, which can inhibit the absorption of many nutrients. Fiber supplements may help relieve constipation, but most health experts advise using food as the primary source of dietary fiber intake. If you feel you need more fiber in your diet through a supplement, talk to your doctor first.

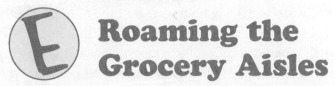

Chapter 5

Roaming the Grocery Aisles

H alf the battle of eating a healthier diet before, during, and after pregnancy is having healthy foods on hand to eat. To have healthier foods on hand, you need to know your way around the grocery store as well as your way around the nutrition facts panel (on all packaged foods). Applying some simple guidelines can help make healthy eating part of your everyday lifestyle.

Before You Shop

The grocery store is packed with aisles and aisles of foods. So where do you start? Your first step should be to do some menu planning. Planning ahead is key to eating healthily and ensuring you get all needed food groups each day. Next, prepare your grocery list from your menus. Hitting the grocery store with a list in your hands will help you resist the impulse to buy those foods you don't need. Don't let your stomach do the shopping!

Set up your shopping list according to the layout of the grocery store where you shop. This will make shopping easier and quicker. When you think of the grocery store layout, most of the fresh foods are on the perimeter of the store, with all other foods in the middle. Start at one end, and work your way around.

Single Out Fruits and Veggies

The produce aisle will provide you and your baby with foods that really pack in the nutrition. Today's stores offer a healthy variety of produce for you to choose from. Fruits and vegetables are naturally low in fat and calories and provide a variety of vitamins, minerals, phytonutrients (plant compounds thought to be beneficial to health), and other essentials. Keeping a stock of fresh fruits and vegetables on hand can make for great snacks and/or tasty additions to your meals. To get your fill of fruits and vegetables each day, try to eat a combination of at least five fruits and vegetables each day.

Produce Shopping Tips

Make your shopping trip interesting and healthy by finding a produce rainbow. Choose fruits and vegetables that span the spectrum from deep red to dark green, yellow, and orange—for instance, spinach, broccoli, carrots, and red peppers. Take full advantage of fruits and vegetables that are in season, which can make them less expensive as well as fresher and more flavorful. When shopping for your produce, always examine it for freshness and ripeness. The fresher the produce, the more nutrients it contains.

It is best to choose fresh or frozen produce over the canned varieties. Canned vegetables can be higher in sodium, and canned fruits can be high in added sugar, so if you do opt for this route, be sure to read the label. Search out varieties that are low in sodium, and rinse the product in a colander before preparing it. For canned fruits, look for brands that are canned in their own juice or packed in 100-percent fruit juice. If you are trying to add more calcium to your diet, choose juices that are fortified with calcium. Because fresh produce is perishable, only buy what you need and will use. If you won't be able to make it back to the store anytime soon, stock up on both fresh and frozen produce. You can use up the fresh first and than have frozen as a backup.

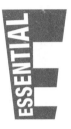

Don't leave dried fruits off your list. They can be very high in fiber and are a great choice during those seasons when the variety of fresh fruit is at a minimum.

What Are Phytochemicals?

Phytochemicals, also known as phytonutrients, are compounds found naturally in plant-based foods—such as fruits, vegetables, legumes, whole grains, nuts, and seeds—that may provide potential health benefits. Phytonutrients are compounds that plants provide naturally to protect themselves against things like viruses, bacteria, and fungi. These phytonutrients are on the cutting edge of health-promoting potential. Though their role is still uncertain, particular phytonutrients may help protect against illnesses including heart disease, certain cancers, high blood pressure, osteoporosis, stroke, cataracts, and other chronic health conditions. There are thousands of phytonutrients—you could find more than 2,000 in the pigments that give plants their color. The more colorful your produce, the more phytonutrients it contains.

Go with the Grain

Whole grains are an important source of the complex carbohydrates that are a major source of energy for both you and the baby. Breads, cereals, rice, and pasta should make up the base of your diet. You will find these in several sections of the grocery store. Grain foods also supply vitamin E, B vitamins such as folic acid, and minerals such as magnesium, iron, and zinc. Whole grains are also rich in fiber.

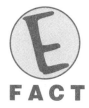

FACT

Whole grains are much more nutritious than refined grains. Refined grains, such as white bread, go through a process that strips them of nutritious parts of the grain. Nutrients such as thiamin, riboflavin, niacin, and folic acid are lost. In some cases the lost nutrients are added back to the product, which are advertised as "enriched." Foods may also be labeled as "fortified," which means that nutrients have been added that were not originally found in the food. For example, some brands of orange juice are fortified with calcium..

When buying bread, read the label to check that whole-wheat flour is the first ingredient listed. If the label specifies whole wheat or whole grain, the bread also contains fiber. Look for bread that provides at least 2 grams of fiber per slice. If you are not a fan of whole-wheat breads, keep in mind that other breads contain fiber, including rye and pumpernickel. Try different brands of whole-wheat bread to find one that you enjoy. When you are shopping for your grain products, look for labels that read "high in fiber" or "good source of fiber." Make your grains count! Choose grain or starch products made with little or no fat and less sugar. In other words, instead of the croissant, go for the whole-wheat bagel. Take advantage of the fiber that cereals can provide. Choose cereals that offer at least 3 grams of fiber, have 3 grams of fat or less, and include 8 grams or less of sugar per serving.

Don't leave out cooked cereal such as oatmeal, grits, or cream of wheat that can be low in fat and high in fiber. Making simple changes, like choosing brown rice over white rice, can pack in a lot more nutrition and fiber.

Brown rice is the only type of whole-grain rice, and it contains more fiber and B vitamins than white rice. Whole-wheat or whole-grain pasta is higher in fiber and B vitamins than regular pasta. Experiment with other grains such as quinoa, millet, or couscous. Get in the habit of looking for the word "whole" in front of grains such as barley, corn, oats, rice, or wheat. Always check the expiration dates on your grain products for freshness. Lastly, keep an eye on various breads like dinner rolls, sandwich bread, or buns—these can pack in the calories unless you pay attention. Check labels for calories per serving.

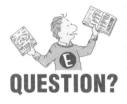

QUESTION?

Are all wheat breads the same?

Just because bread is labeled "wheat" or "multigrain" or because it is brown in color does not necessarily mean it is high in fiber or even that it has fiber at all. In some breads, the brown color comes from caramel coloring, which must be included in the ingredient list. By law, bread labeled "whole wheat" must be made from 100-percent whole-wheat flour. Bread labeled simply as "wheat" can include both wheat and refined white flour, and proportions vary from product to product.

Delectable Dairy

We all know how important calcium is to healthy bones for mother and baby. Supplied mostly by the dairy group, calcium is also usually accompanied by other important nutrients including protein, vitamin D, riboflavin, phosphorus, potassium, and vitamin A. The dairy group includes milk, yogurt, cheese, cottage cheese, and even favorites such as ice cream and frozen yogurt. Because they are an animal source, dairy foods can also contribute to saturated fat and cholesterol intake, so choosing lower-fat or fat-free versions of these foods can help keep your levels down. Skim milk has all the important nutrients in the same quantity as low-fat or whole milk.

The dairy aisle is a vast wilderness of milk, yogurt, cheese, cottage cheese, and many other products. To make sure you get the nutrients you need without too many calories and saturated fat, choose low-fat or fat-free milk, yogurt, cheese, and cottage cheese. Low-fat cheese has 3 grams or less of fat per serving. Cheeses that are made with low-fat milk are also lower in fat, such as part-skim mozzarella. Yogurt is a wonderful food, but fruited yogurts tend to range widely in calorie and fat content, so it is important to check the nutrition facts panel. For optimal freshness, look for the sell-by date (the last date on which the food should be sold) on dairy foods. If lactose intolerance is a problem for you, look for lactose-reduced or lactose-free milk and other dairy products. Soy milk is lactose free, but make sure the brand you choose is fortified with calcium.

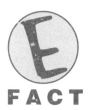

FACT

Cottage cheese has less calcium than other dairy products because during processing, the whey, which contains 50 to 75 percent of the calcium, is drained away. Look for cottage cheese products that are processed with extra calcium. Cottage cheese still contains plenty of protein and riboflavin and little fat.

Protein Power Foods

This group includes meats, poultry, fish, dry beans, eggs, and nuts. Most of these foods you will find in the fresh meat, seafood, and deli cases. This group supplies large amounts of protein as well as other essential nutrients including zinc, iron, and B vitamins. The meat group can also be a large source of saturated fat and cholesterol, so it is important to choose lean cuts.

Choosing Meats Wisely

Protein foods that come from animal sources can be confusing when it comes to fat content, so it is important to choose wisely. Choose leaner cuts of beef, which you can usually tell by their names: "round" cuts, such as eye of round or round roast, or "loin" cuts, such as tenderloin or sirloin. Other lean cuts include the flank (such as flank steak), porterhouse steak or roast, and T-bone steak. For leaner cuts of pork, chose a name that includes "loin," such as loin chop or tenderloin.

With seafood, meat, or poultry, look for labels marked "lean." This means that each 3-ounce serving includes the following:

- Less than 10 grams of total fat
- 4 grams of saturated fat
- 95 mg cholesterol

For products marked "extra lean," a 3-ounce serving includes:

- Less than 5 grams total fat
- 2 grams saturated fat
- 95 mg cholesterol

When it comes to ground beef, stick to leaner varieties. Ground beef that is 95 percent lean meets government standards for "lean." Ground round is the leanest ground beef followed by ground sirloin, ground chuck, then regular ground meat. Beef is graded by the U.S. Department of Agriculture based on fat content, appearance, texture, and age of the animal. The "Select" grade has the least amount of marbled fat, which is followed by "Choice," then "Prime" cuts of beef. Prime cuts are the juiciest and most flavorful, but they also contain the most fat. With proper cooking techniques, Select and Choice cuts can be just as tender and juicy as Prime cuts. Pork is not graded.

Many ground meats now have labels, so if you are not sure about the fat content, compare the labels of different cuts. Always buy meat that is well trimmed, with no more than an eighth of an inch of visible fat trim. Trim refers to the fat layer surrounding the cut of meat. Marbled fat is the fat within the meat that shows as white streaks throughout the piece of meat. Marbled fat can't be trimmed, but with the correct cooking methods it can be somewhat decreased. Check packages of meat to find the highest lean-to-fat ratio. Ensure that meat is fresh by checking out the color. Beef is typically bright red, young veal and pork are grayish-pink, and older veal is a darker pink. Check the dates on meat also because with some meat items, such as ground beef, exposure to oxygen even under plastic wrap can cause the outer layer of the meat to darken.

What to Know About Poultry

Poultry is a bit leaner than some red meats, but it is still important to know some essential tips. Choose leaner varieties of poultry such as chicken and turkey, and choose skinless to make it easier to trim fat before cooking. If buying poultry with skin, remove the skin before cooking. Try ground turkey for a leaner alternative to ground beef. Be sure the ground turkey package states "lean" or "very lean," which means it is made from white-meat turkey. The fat content is higher if it is ground with dark meat and skin.

If you're buying a whole turkey, keep in mind that self-basting varieties are usually higher in fat because they are injected with fat to help preserve moisture. For freshness, check dates and look for meaty poultry with skin that is creamy white to yellow and that is free of bruises, tiny feathers, and torn or dry skin. Also check the nutrition facts panel. Some of these foods may not be as low in fat as you assume, and some may be high in sodium.

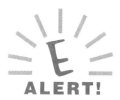

ALERT!

Lean-to-fat ratios on ground meat can vary greatly. On a package of ground meat, the term "percent lean" refers to the weight of the meat in relation to the weight of the fat in the meat. Therefore, in a package of 95-percent lean ground beef, fat accounts for 5 percent of the weight of the meat. The 95 percent lean ground beef is the only cut of ground beef that meets the government's labeling guidelines for "lean."

Fish Facts

Fish can be a wonderful source of some very healthy fats. Buy fish only from a reputable source, and make sure the fish or seafood is stored properly in the refrigerator or freezer. Most fish has less fat than meat or poultry, and most of the fat from fish is a polyunsaturated source (a healthy fat) such as omega-3 fatty acid. Fattier fish has more omega-3 fatty acids than lean fish or shellfish, and these fats may offer heart-healthy benefits. Fish that is white or light in color such as perch, orange roughy, snapper, and sole is lower in fat than fish that is firm and darker in color, such as mackerel and salmon. Always check the dates on fish to make sure it is fresh, and for safety do not buy cooked seafood that is displayed alongside raw fish or seafood. Breaded fish can be higher in fat and calories. Consider buying fresh fish and breading it and baking it yourself.

The "Others"

In addition to meat, poultry, and fish, there are other foods in this group to take a look at, such as eggs. Egg yolks contain a significant amount of fat and cholesterol. The refrigerated egg substitutes available at your grocery store offer a cholesterol-free and lower-fat option. Always check the expiration date on eggs for freshness.

This food group also includes plant-based foods, including dried beans, peas, and lentils, which are excellent sources of protein and fiber. Choose these as an alternative to meat a few times a week and add them to salads, casseroles, soups, or stews. Soy products such as tofu, soy milk, and veggie burgers can also be an excellent source of protein, and they also make a good alternative to meat occasionally. They are low in fat, contain no cholesterol, and are good sources of fiber.

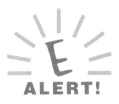
ALERT!

If you follow a strict vegan diet (that is, you eat no foods of any animal origin), you still need to ensure that you consume plenty of protein as well as the other nutrients that this food group supplies. Your doctor may prescribe additional supplements, and a dietitian can help you devise a well-balanced eating plan. See Chapter 9 for additional information.

Figuring Fats

Foods high in fat, such as oils, salad dressings, cream, butter, gravy, and margarine, need to be used sparingly. For most of the foods in this category, it is best to choose lower-fat versions. They add flavor to foods and can be part of a healthy diet if consumed in moderation. Keep in mind that fat-free foods are not necessarily calorie-free, or even low calorie. Nonstick cooking sprays can take the place of oils for cooking or baking, which saves on calories.

When purchasing fats, remember to stick to predominantly unsaturated fats, which are the healthy fats. Soft margarines or tub margarines are healthier choices because they don't contain as much saturated fat and/or trans-fatty acids as stick margarines. Avoid those listing hydrogenated or partially hydrogenated fat as the first ingredient. Look for new margarine products that are free from trans-fatty acids or hydrogenated fats. These fats can increase blood cholesterol just as much as saturated fat and dietary cholesterol.

Convenience Items

There are all kinds of foods available that can help make meals more convenient. These convenience foods range from frozen meals to canned soups to boxed meals. While you're still in the grocery store, be sure you read the nutrition facts panels. Be aware of the fat, sodium, calories, and other nutrients these foods provide. Don't swap convenience for good nutrition. Use the nutrition facts panel to compare frozen meals and entrees. Choose ones that are lower in calories, fat, saturated fat, cholesterol, and sodium. Experts advise you to choose those frozen entrées with less than 15 grams of fat, 300 to 400 calories, and 600 to 800 mg sodium. Keep in mind that many frozen meals typically lack fruit, vegetables, and calcium. To consume a more complete meal, supplement these meals with whole foods.

Many convenience foods can be higher in sodium. If you are watching your sodium intake, read the nutrition facts panel to keep track of their sodium content. Many canned and instant soups are high in sodium, so look for soups prepared with less. Boxed meals can also be a high-sodium product, so choose those that are lower in sodium and fat. Many times, you can prepare boxed items in such a way as to lower their fat or sodium contents, such as by using fat-free milk or using half of the seasoning packet provided.

Reading the Food Label

The grocery store is full of thousands of food items, giving you at least that many choices. You need to be armed with information and education in order to make smarter choices, and that means knowing and understanding the food label. The information included on this label gives you the freedom to compare products and choose ones that best fits your nutritional needs. It is well worth your time and effort to learn how to interpret food labels and how to put them to work for you and your baby. The major parts of the food label include the nutrition facts panel, the ingredient list, health claims, and nutritional claims.

The Nutrition Facts Panel

At the very top of the nutrition facts panel is the serving size, the number of servings included in the container, the calories per serving, and the number and percentage of calories that come from fat. Below that is a list of the three macronutrients (fat, carbohydrates, and protein) as well as other important nutrients. These nutrients are listed in grams or milligrams. Below those are listed a few micronutrients, two vitamins and two minerals, which are displayed in percentages. On the right side of the panel is a column headed "% Daily Value." Near the bottom of the panel is the statement that the percent daily values are based on a 2,000-calorie diet, as well as a list of daily reference values.

FIGURE 3-1
Nutrition
facts panel

Servings per container refer to the number of servings found in this container.

Amount per serving refers to the nutrient content for each serving of food.

This section lists the recommended daily limits of fat, saturated fat, cholesterol, and sodium, plus amounts of carbohydrates and fiber one should aim for on a daily basis for diets of 2,000 and 2,500 calories.

Nutrition Facts

Serving Size 1/2 cup (114 g)
Servings Per Container 4

Amount Per Serving

Calories: 90   Calories from Fat 30

% Daily Value*

Total Fat 3g	5%
Saturated Fat 0g	0%
Cholesterol 0mg	0%
Sodium 300mg	13%
Total Carbohydrate 13g	4%
Dietary Fiber 3g	12%
Sugars 3g	
Protein 3g	

Vitamin A 80%	Vitamin C 60%
Calcium 4% •	Iron 4%

* Percent Daily Values are based on a 2,000-calorie diet. Your daily values may be higher or lower depending on your calorie needs:

	Calories: 2,000	2,500
Total Fat	Less than 65g	80g
Saturated Fat	Less than 20g	25g
Cholesterol	Less than 300g	300g
Sodium	Less than 2,400mg	2,400mg
Total Carbohydrate	300mg	375mg
Dietary Fiber	25g	30g

Calories per gram
Fat 9 • Carbohydrate 4 • Protein 4

The **serving size** refers to the average amount or portion a person should eat at one time.

% Daily Value is based on a 2,000-calorie daily diet. These values may be higher or lower based on the number of calories in one's diet. One should aim for 100% each day of total carbohydrate, dietary fiber, vitamins, and minerals and not exceed 100% for total fat, sodium and cholesterol.

Serving Size

The serving size is extremely important because everything on the panel pertains to the specified serving size. The serving size refers to the average amount or portion a person should eat at one time. On the sample panel, the serving size is ½ cup, and there are four servings per container. So, all of the information on the panel pertains to ½ cup serving. If you ate the whole container, you would need to multiply the information on the panel by four.

Counting Calories

The panel provides information on how many calories there are in a single serving of the particular food. The panel also provides you with the number of calories that come from fat in one serving. In the example panel, there are 90 calories in a serving and 30 calories come from fat. This means that out of the total 90 calories per serving, 30, or one-third, of them are coming from fat. We know that calories in food only come from three sources: fat, protein, and carbohydrate. So this also tells you that the other 60 calories come from protein and/or carbohydrate sources. When reading a panel, it is important to consider all of the other foods you eat during the day. One food may contribute more calories or nutrients than others, but it won't provide your total nutritional intake for the day.

Nutrients on the Panel

The specific nutrients that are listed on the nutrition facts panel were selected by the USDA and the FDA because of their relationship to current health issues. Nutrients that are required on all food labels include total fat, saturated fat, cholesterol, sodium, total carbohydrate, dietary fiber, sugar, protein, vitamin A, vitamin C, calcium, and iron. Manufacturers can list additional nutrients, but only these are required.

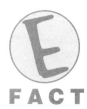

FACT

The total fat content consists of both types of fat: saturated and unsaturated (polyunsaturated and monounsaturated). The label must also list saturated fat content; unsaturated can be listed but is not required.

The first four nutrients that are listed represent those that Americans generally consume in excess (fat, saturated fat, cholesterol, and sodium). The two vitamins and two minerals displayed on the panel are listed as reference to the reference daily intakes (RDIs). The RDIs are values established by the FDA that are used only on food labels.

The RDI for the two vitamins and two minerals required on every food label are the following:

- Vitamin A—5,000 international units (IU)
- Vitamin C—60 mg
- Calcium—1,000 mg
- Iron—18 mg

For example, if a label states that a product contains 50 percent of the RDI of vitamin A, it contains 2,500 IUs. Keep in mind that RDIs are relevant for the "average" person. Women who are pregnant may have higher needs, and you should pay attention to your specific nutrient needs. Use the food label not only to help limit those nutrients you should cut back on but also to increase those nutrients and other things you should consume more of, such as vitamins, minerals, and fiber.

Percent Daily Value

The percent daily value is the most misunderstood part of the panel. The nutrients on food labels are expressed in two distinct ways. First, as explained above, they are expressed in terms of the amount by weight (in grams or milligrams) per serving. The other way these nutrients are expressed is in terms of percent daily value. This measure gives an estimate of how a serving of a particular food meets the daily requirement for each nutrient, based on a 2,000-calorie diet. Daily reference values, or the amounts of nutrients you should get for a healthy diet, based on a 2,000-calorie diet, are shown on the bottom of each panel underneath the vitamin/mineral information. For example, if a panel states that the product contains 5 percent of the daily value for fat, one serving of that food product will give 5 percent of the 65 grams (or 3 grams) you are allowed for the day on a 2,000-calorie diet.

Using Percent Daily Value

This information is meant to help you decide whether a specific nutrient in a serving of food contributes a lot or a little to your total daily intake. Your goal each day should be to meet 100 percent or less of the daily value for nutrients you should be consuming less of, such as fat, saturated fat, sodium, sugar, and cholesterol. Likewise, your goal should be to get 100 percent or more for nutrients and other things you should be consuming more of, such as fiber, com plex carbohydrates, calcium, iron, vitamin A, and vitamin C. Keep in mind that during pregnancy, your caloric goal will most likely be more than 2,000 calories per day. If you should be consuming more than 2,000 calories, the percent daily value can be adjusted for your specific calorie level.

To determine the proper adjustment of the percent daily value for you, first calculate your estimated basic calorie needs (as described in Chapter 3, on page 33). Match that number against the numbers in the left-hand column of the following table. Then check the right-hand column to see how to adjust the percent daily values. For instance, a woman who needs 2,500 calories to maintain her weight would adjust the percent daily values by 125 percent, meaning that she should consume 25 percent more of those nutrients than the amounts listed on the panels.

Calories	Adjusted % Daily Value
2,000	100 percent
2,200	110 percent
2,500	125 percent
2,800	140 percent
3,200	160 percent

The percent daily value can help you quickly decide whether a food is high or low in a particular nutrient. A food is considered low in a nutrient if one serving contains 5 percent or less of that nutrient's daily value. Descriptive words that are used on panels to describe low nutrient levels include "few," "contains a small amount of," "low source of," "low in," "little," and "a little." A food is a good source of a particular nutrient if one serving contains 10 to 19 percent of the daily value for a nutrient. Other terms that can be used to fit this definition include "contains" and "provides." A food is considered high in a nutrient if one serving contains 20 percent or more of the daily value for a particular nutrient. Panels describe high nutrient levels with terms such as "excellent source of" and "rich in."

Calculating Percent Daily Value

The reference daily values shown on each panel are calculated using the following nutritional recommendations.

Nutrient	Recommended Levels*
Total fat	30 percent of total calories
Saturated fat	10 percent of total calories
Total carbohydrate	60 percent of total calories
Fiber**	11.5 grams per 1,000 calories
Cholesterol***	Less than 300 mg per day
Sodium***	Less than 2,400 mg per day
Potassium (optional)	3,500 mg per day

*Some numbers are rounded off for nutrition labeling.

**20 grams is the minimum amount of fiber recommended for all calorie levels below 2,000.

***Recommended cholesterol and sodium levels are always constant no matter how many calories are consumed.

The percent daily value is helpful when it comes to menu planning because it helps you see your intake of various nutrients in relation to the reference daily value instead of as a simple quantitative value. For example, a food that contains 150 mg of sodium could seem high in sodium just because the number 150 seems large. In actuality, however, 150 mg is only about 6 percent of the daily value for sodium of 2,400 mg per day. On the other hand, a food with 5 grams of saturated fat could be construed as being low in that nutrient because five is a small number. But in reality, that food provides 25 percent of the total daily value for saturated fat (20 grams).

Label Claims

Labels often contain both nutrition and health claims. Nutrition claims or nutrition descriptions can help you to quickly and easily find foods that meet your specific nutritional goals. These include claims such as "high calcium," "low fat," "cholesterol free," "high fiber," and "low sodium." Nutrition claims are not required on labels. Regulations by the FDA strictly spell out what terms may be used to describe the level of a specific nutrient in a food and how they can be used. Some of the general claims used include "free," "low," "light," "more," and "reduced."

Specific definitions of claims for particular nutrients include the following.

Claim	What It Means
Low fat	3 g or less per serving
Low in saturated fat	1 g or less per serving
Low sodium	140 mg or less per serving
Very low sodium	35 mg or less per serving
Low cholesterol	20 mg or less, and 2 g or less of saturated fat per serving
Low calorie	40 calories or less per serving

Health claims describe potential health benefits of a specific food or nutrient provided by the food. You have read or heard advertising that claims calcium is of benefit in reducing osteoporosis, or that folic acid is helpful in reducing the risk of neural tube birth defects. Health claims are not required to be included on labels. If they are included, however, health claims on packaged foods must also be approved and must be scientifically validated by the FDA. All of these claims must use the phrasing "may" or "might" help prevent.

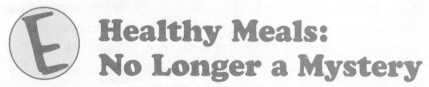

Chapter 6

Healthy Meals: No Longer a Mystery

Healthy meals don't have to be a mystery! A little extra planning, a few modifications, and the right choices can make all the difference. Knowing what to do (and what not to do) in the kitchen is essential. Nor does eating out have to mean eating unhealthy foods. Use this chapter to help you unlock the mystery and make healthy meals part of your everyday lifestyle.

Planning the Family Menu

Planning meals for yourself usually means planning meals for the whole family. The best way to make sure you and your family eat a healthy diet is to plan ahead. Plan menus for the week, and make sure you have all the foods necessary to carry out your plan. Planning ahead can help deter haphazard eating, which can lead to overeating or eating the wrong foods, and it helps you to stock your kitchen with the right ingredients.

Good menu planning is based on the right balance of foods. That means using the food groups and making sure you get enough of what you need at each meal to reach your goal for the day. Plan to eat five to six small meals throughout the day. This helps to keep your energy levels stable from meal to meal and gives you more opportunities to fit in all the food groups that you need.

Benefits of Planning Ahead

There are many benefits to planning ahead that can help both your nutritional intake as well as your busy lifestyle. Dinner can be a much less hectic event when you know what the menu will be in advance. By planning ahead, you can make meal preparation less time-consuming, and your family will probably tend to eat together more frequently. Planning ahead also sends you to the grocery store with a list, which can help you to avoid impulse purchases at the grocery store (and thus saving you some money!). When you plan meals, you don't tend to eat out or order out as much, which can be costly to both your pocketbook and your daily food intake.

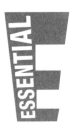

Build some flexibility into your weekly menu plan in case things don't go as planned, which can happen at any time! Once you plan a week of menus, keep them around and recycle them down the road.

Steps to Easy Meal Planning

Menu planning does not have to be a complicated task. A small investment of your time can reap great rewards. Menu plans can save you money by cutting out the need for last-minute trips to the grocery store. Most important, planning ahead helps conserve your most valuable resource: your energy. You don't need to plan for the next month; just plan for the next week. Keep staple foods on hand for healthy breakfasts and snacks, and then decide on a few lunches that you can eat a few times during the week. That leaves you with just seven simple dinners to plan.

Think of dishes that can be used for leftovers the next night—for instance, a pan of lasagna is sure to last you a few nights. Do your meal planning on the days that your local grocery store ads come out; this can help give you ideas for dinners for the week and will let you know which foods are on special. To come up with some ideas of meals to prepare, get out your favorite recipes or cookbooks, and see what you already have on hand. Plan meals according to your and your family's schedule, for instance, by saving the roast for a lazy Sunday and preparing a homemade pizza on the day when the kids have soccer and you work late.

Mastering Low-Fat Cooking

While planning your meals, think healthy. The methods that you use to prepare your meals can make a big difference in the amount of calories, total fat, saturated fat, and cholesterol content they contain. With a few simple changes and tips to cooking methods, you can cook "leaner" and still have great-tasting dishes. Use cooking methods that require little fat, such as braising, broiling, grilling, pan-broiling, poaching, roasting, simmering, steaming, stewing, and stir-frying. Simply trimming visible fat and skin from poultry) before cooking can cut fat significantly. If you leave the skin on while cooking, remove it before eating.

Other tips include running ground meat in hot water after browning and then draining to rinse off excess fat. You can also pat the meat with a paper towel or drain on a paper towel to remove excess fat. For meat that has little to no fat, try using marinades such as teriyaki sauce, orange juice, lime juice, lemon juice, tomato juice, defatted broth, or low-fat yogurt. Add fresh herbs and other spices, such as garlic powder, to marinades for more flavors. Did you ever notice that fat collects on top of stew, soups, chili, or other casserole dishes? Chill these dishes overnight, and the fat will rise to the top, making it easy for you to skim off. If you are not afraid to experiment, use half meat and half tofu, tempeh, or legumes to lower the fat in recipes and increase fiber. Stock your kitchen with nonstick saucepans, skillets, and baking pans so you can sauté and bake without adding additional fat. If you need to, use a nonstick cooking spray along with defatted broth, water, juice, or cooking wine to replace cooking oil and prevent sticking.

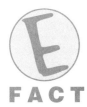

FACT

Grilling can be a great low-fat cooking method, but it does have a few downsides. Recent research has indicated that potential carcinogens (cancer-causing substances) may be present in grilled foods. To make grilled food safer, do not char meats or vegetables, use a low to medium heat, reduce time on the grill by baking or microwaving foods first, and avoid eating the blackened parts of grilled foods.

Healthy-Up Your Recipes

In addition to using healthier cooking techniques, swapping ingredients in your recipes for leaner ones can healthy-up your meals. Small changes within a recipe can make big difference in the nutritional outcome. You may need to use less of an ingredient, substitute an ingredient, add a new ingredient, or completely leave something out. It will take some trial and error to get your recipes to your liking, but the extra effort will be well worth it.

Take a look at your recipes before you get started, and think about what individual ingredients may contribute to a dish that's higher in fat, cholesterol, calories, or sodium. Decide which ingredients can be substituted or reduced as well as added for additional nutritional value. Adding shredded carrots or zucchini to your lasagna, for example, can add a load of extra vitamins, minerals, and fiber to your dish. Make changes to your recipes gradually by changing one or two ingredients at a time each time you make it.

Use some of these substitutions to cut fat and calories while cooking or baking:

- Use fat-free or low-fat milk instead of whole milk.
- Use low-fat yogurt, ½ cup cottage cheese blended with 1½ teaspoon lemon juice, or light or fat-free sour cream instead of regular sour cream.
- Use evaporated fat-free milk or fat-free half-and-half instead of cream.
- Use 3 tablespoons cocoa powder plus 1 tablespoon oil instead of 1 ounce unsweetened baking chocolate.
- Use low-fat cottage cheese or low-fat or nonfat ricotta cheese instead of regular ricotta cheese.
- Use chocolate sauce instead of fudge sauce.
- Use nonfat or low-fat plain yogurt or reduced-fat mayonnaise instead of regular mayonnaise.
- Use pureed fruits such as applesauce to replace anywhere from a third to half of the fat in recipes.
- For pies and other desserts, use a graham-cracker crumb crust instead of a higher-fat pastry shell.
- Use pureed cooked vegetables instead of cream, egg yolks, or roux to thicken sauces and soups.

Sensible Snacking

Choosing healthy snacks is as important as the healthy meals that you plan. Healthy snacks can help you add those extra calories and nutrients you need during pregnancy as well as give you a boost of energy when you need it and take the edge off hunger in between meals. Contrary to popular belief, snacking can be part of a healthful eating plan. To keep blood sugar levels under control, it is ideal to go no longer than three or four hours between meals. The key to sensible snacking is the type and amount of food that you choose. Mindless snacking or nibbling on high-fat, high-calorie foods can lead to trouble in the form of unwanted and empty calories as well as loads of fat and sugar.

To make snacking a healthy part of your diet, choose snacks that are lower in fat and rich in nutrients. Make snacks count, instead of thinking of them as an "extra." Eat snacks well ahead of mealtime, and eat smaller portions of your snacks as opposed to big ones. Also, plan your snacks ahead of time. Good snack ideas include the following:

- Half a whole-wheat bagel or an apple topped with peanut butter
- Celery stalks with low-fat cream cheese
- Low-fat fruited yogurt topped with low-fat granola cereal
- Low-fat cottage cheese topped with fresh fruit
- Fresh fruit
- Light microwave popcorn (for extra flavor, toss with a small amount of low-fat Parmesan cheese or garlic powder)
- Pita bread stuffed with fresh veggies and low-fat ranch dressing
- Low-fat string cheese and crackers
- Raisins and rice cakes

These are only a few ideas! Use your creativity, and choose foods that you like.

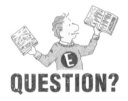

QUESTION?

Can eating more than three times a day be part of a healthy diet?
Yes. For women who are pregnant or for anybody who enjoys a healthy lifestyle, eating several small meals during the day can fit nicely into a healthy eating pattern. It can help you to fit in those extra calories and food group servings without having to eat large meals all at once, which can be difficult for women who may be having a problem with nausea or morning sickness.

Portion Power

Portion sizes are very important when you're trying to eat a healthy diet and control your calorie intake. The portion sizes you consume contribute directly to the number of calories and the amount of fat and other nutrients that you consume per day. Don't forget that even though you need a few more calories while pregnant, you are still not eating for two adult people.

You can eat healthily and still be eating too much. To follow the guidelines of the Food Guide Pyramid correctly, you must be aware of the portion sizes that you eat.

Visualize Your Portions

To follow a healthy diet, you don't need to necessarily weigh and measure all of your food each day. But you do need a general idea of how much you should be eating. Keep in mind that portion sizes are meant as general guidelines—the goal is to come close to the recommended serving sizes on average over several days. Be careful of letting your stomach do the portioning. Skipping meals can lead to ravenous hunger at the next meal, which makes it difficult to correctly portion your foods. To help estimate your portion sizes, use these visual comparisons:

- A 3-ounce portion of cooked meat, poultry, or fish is about the size of a deck of playing cards.
- A medium potato is about the size of a computer mouse.
- One cup of rice or pasta is about the size of a fist or a tennis ball.
- An average bagel should be the size of a hockey puck or a large to-go coffee lid.
- A cup of fruit or a medium apple or orange is the size of a baseball.
- One-half cup of chopped vegetables is about the size of three regular ice cubes.
- Three ounces of grilled fish is the size of your checkbook.
- One ounce of cheese is the size of four dice.
- One teaspoon of peanut butter equals one dice, and two tablespoons is about the size of a golf ball.
- One ounce of snack foods—such as pretzels—equals a large handful.
- A thumb tip equals 1 teaspoon, three thumb tips equal 1 tablespoon and a whole thumb equals 1 ounce.

To help you eat only the portions you measure out, portion out your food before bringing it to the table. You will be less likely to eat too much when serving bowls are not on the table. Another clever trick is to use a smaller plate to make your portion sizes look bigger.

Dining Out

It is nice to get out of the kitchen once in awhile and let someone else do the cooking. According to the National Restaurant Association, in 2000, the average annual household expenditure away from home was about $855 per person. About half of all adults eat at a restaurant on a typical day, and almost 54 billion meals are eaten in restaurants, at school, and at work cafeterias each year. But dining out can present challenges to your goal of eating healthily during your pregnancy.

The more meals that are eaten away from home, the bigger impact they have on your total daily nutritional intake. It is much easier to splurge or lose sight of your overall eating pattern when you eat out frequently. All of this eating out generates nutritional challenges that include larger-than-normal portion sizes, too many calories, too much fat and sodium, too few vitamins and minerals, and too little fiber.

Your Dining-Out Guidelines

Even though dining out can present some challenges, this doesn't mean you can't eat out occasionally. It simply means that you have to put some thought into the choices that you make when dining out. It also means that you will have to put a greater effort to balance out the rest of your day's intake. When you are at a restaurant, be the first to order your meal so you are not tempted by what other people order. Make an effort to eat slowly and stop eating before you feel too stuffed. You can ask the server to remove your plate once you feel full. If there is food left on your plate, ask for a doggie bag. Try splitting a meal with a dining companion, or bring half your meal home in a doggie bag for lunch the next day. In fact, you can even ask for a doggie bag to come with your meal so you can pack half of it away and not be tempted to eat the whole thing.

Start with easy changes, like choosing low-calorie salad dressings. You can also ask for dressing, gravies, sauces, and condiments (like mayonnaise) to be served on the side. This way, you have more control over how much you use. Small changes can go a long way. Don't be afraid to ask exactly how foods are prepared or to ask to have them prepared in a certain way. When choosing entrees, opt for plain meats and vegetables instead of breaded and/or deep-fried dishes, and avoid sauces and ingredients such as hollandaise, butter, cheese, and cream sauces that can add extra calories and fat.

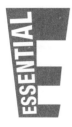

Menu terms that are clues to lower-fat foods include the following words: baked, braised, broiled, grilled, roasted, steamed, stir-fried, poached, or cooked in its own juices. Menu clues that a food is likely to be higher in fat include these: alfredo, au gratin, cheese sauce, battered, fried, béarnaise, buttered, creamed, French fried, hollandaise, pan fried, sautéed, scalloped, with gravy, or with sauce. Menu clues that a food may be higher in sodium include these words: barbecued, in broth, pickled, smoked, teriyaki, Creole sauce, or soy sauce.

Request substitutes for higher-fat side dishes. For example, if your meal comes with French fries, ask for a baked potato with salsa, a brothy soup, side salad, or fresh fruit bowl instead. Be careful of appetizers before your meal that can really add up in fat and calories. Instead, choose fresh fruit, vegetable juice, marinated vegetables, raw vegetables with salsa dip, or seafood cocktail. Be very careful of beverages such as alcohol and soft drinks that can add tons of empty calories to your meal. You best bet is water with a twist of lemon—and keep it coming, especially if you're trying to avoid the bread basket! Most importantly, balance your dining-out habits with physical activity. Being physically active is what helps burn those calories. After you get home from eating out, take a walk.

Plan for Dining Out

Planning ahead for a meal out can put you on the right path to a healthier eating experience. Plan your day so that you can fit the restaurant meal into your whole day's eating plan. Nutritional intake is what you take in over the course of an entire day, not just one meal. Never skip meals during the day just to "save up" for your night out. If you arrive at the restaurant ravenous, you will probably eat more than you intended to, and you will probably have a harder time making healthier choices. Instead, eat light meals throughout the day, and have a snack such as yogurt or fruit in the late afternoon. Choosing a restaurant that prepares foods to order will help give you more control of what you eat and will make it easier to make special requests. This means passing up the all-you-can-eat buffets. Do some homework, and call ahead to a restaurant you plan to visit to ask about the menu and how food is prepared.

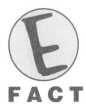

FACT

An order of twelve buffalo wings can weigh in at up to 700 calories and 48 grams. An order of eight stuffed potato skins with sour cream can add up to 1,260 calories and 95 grams of fat. A fried onion bloom (serving size of three cups) with dipping sauce can add up to 2,130 calories and 163 grams of fat. Plan on skipping the appetizer and just going straight to the healthy meal.

Obstacles at the Salad Bar

The salad bar always seems like a safe bet, but be aware that it can be a pitfall of excessive calories and fat if you are not careful. Choosing a large variety of vegetables and fruits can add to your day's intake of essential vitamins, minerals, and fiber. However, depending on what foods you choose, your salad bar plate can still add up to 1,000 calories or more. Excessive calories at the salad bar usually come from regular salad dressings, cheese, bacon bits, croutons, nuts or seeds, olives, and other side dishes such as macaroni salad, pasta salad, creamy soups, and even desserts. To help control your trip to the salad bar and make it a healthy one, use plenty of fresh vegetables as the base of your salad. By choosing dark-green leafy lettuces, such as romaine and/or spinach, over iceberg lettuce, you can add more essential vitamins, minerals, and fiber. Stick with lower-fat or fat-free salad dressings if you tend to eat a little salad with your dressing. Add protein to your salad plate by adding lean meats such as turkey, chicken breast, or egg whites; legumes such as chickpeas; or crabmeat. Add low-fat cottage cheese, other low-fat cheeses, and yogurt to add a calcium boost. Go easy on those mayonnaise-based salads, such as potato or macaroni salad, that always seem to be there, and stick to fresh fruits for dessert.

Fumbling for Fast Food

How many times have you been out running around—or home but not in the mood to do any cooking—and decided to stop at the first fast-food place you saw? Fast foods are more popular than ever before, and many now offer a variety of healthy menu alternatives. Still, frequenting fast-food places can lead to a higher intake of fat, calories, sodium, saturated fat, and cholesterol. It can also cut into your chances of getting in all the food groups you need each day, including fruits, vegetables, dairy, and whole grains. Some pregnant women may lose their taste altogether for that fast-food burger, while others may begin to crave them.

When choosing your fast-food entrée, choose smaller burgers without the cheese, bacon, mayonnaise, and special sauces. All these toppers add more saturated fat and cholesterol to your meal, not to mention calories. Use lower-fat toppings such as ketchup, mustard, barbeque sauces, lettuce, tomatoes, and pickles. Better yet, go for the grilled chicken breast or a sensible salad. If you choose to eat chicken or fish, stay away from the deep-fried versions, which will be high in fat and calories. A grilled, roasted, or broiled piece of chicken or fish is the healthiest choice.

Toppings can add up quickly, as follows:

- One packet of mayonnaise can have as much as 95 calories and 10 grams of fat.
- One packet of tartar sauce can add as much as 160 calories and 17 grams of fat to your fish sandwich.
- A 2-ounce packet of ranch dressing can have as much as 290 calories and 30 grams of fat.
- Just one slice of American cheese can add 50 calories and 5 grams of fat.

Subs can make for a healthy, low-fat sandwich when prepared on whole-grain bread and topped with mustard, vegetable oil, and/or low-fat cheese. Go for the cooked turkey or chicken breast instead of the higher-fat processed meats such as salami or bologna. Load up your sub with vegetables such as lettuce, tomato, onions, and peppers. Wraps are also a good choice. These are usually made from pita bread or flour tortillas and stuffed with chicken, beans, and/or vegetables. Again, beware of the added cheese, dressings, and sauces that can turn a simple sub into a high-fat and high-calorie nightmare. Ask for half the cheese, and ask for the dressing and sauce on the side so you can choose a lower-fat or fat-free version.

Not sure how your favorite fast-food menus rate? Most fast-food restaurants have Web sites that post nutritional information on their foods. Check them out before you head off to the drive-through!

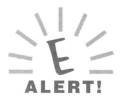

ALERT!

We're a country of people who love our French fries. But don't be fooled into thinking this is a health food now that fast-food restaurants are telling us their fries are fried in vegetable oil. These oils are hydrogenated to make them more solid at room temperature, which means they are loaded with saturated fat. The best choice for a side dish is a garden salad with low-fat or fat-free dressing or a baked potato loaded with salsa.

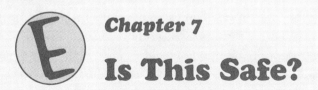

Chapter 7

Is This Safe?

Now that you are pregnant, you want to make sure that everything you put in your mouth is safe for you and your baby. There are many different products that fall into this group, including everything from food additives to medications. Let this chapter guide you through some of the questions you may have.

Exploring Food Additives

Many of the foods we eat are chock-full of food additives such as preservatives, flavor enhancers, food colorings, and even hormones. These additives are used to add color, flavor, enhance flavor, sweeten, and preserve food freshness. New additives must pass very rigid government safety tests before they are considered safe for consumers. The U.S. Food and Drug Administration (FDA) is the entity responsible for approving additives used in foods. The FDA sets safety standards, determines whether a substance is safe for its intended use, decides what type of foods the additive can be used in, what amounts it can be used in, and how it must be indicated on food labels.

Regulating Additives

Some additives are labeled as "Generally recognized as safe" (GRAS) because they have an extensive history of safe use or because existing scientific evidence indicates their safe use in foods. There is an extensive list of GRAS additives, which the FDA and USDA re-evaluate from time to time.

Additives fall into three categories: prior-approved substances, regulated additives, and color additives. Prior-approved substances are additives that were approved prior to the 1958 Food Additives Amendment, which made the FDA responsible for approving additives. Regulated additives are not considered as GRAS or prior-approved until they are fully approved and go through rigorous testing. Before color additives can be used in food, they need to be tested the same as regulated food additives.

Most food additives are safe during pregnancy unless you have a known reaction or specific allergy to certain food additives. As a pregnant woman, you should get in the habit of reading labels carefully, especially if you are sensitive to any food additives or colorings. If you are concerned about food additives, the best advice is to eat a wide variety of fresh foods. A diet high in whole grains, fresh fruits, fresh vegetables, and fresh meats can help you avoid excessive amounts of some food additives.

MSG

Monosodium glutamate, known as MSG, is used as a flavor enhancer. MSG does not add a flavor of its own to food; instead, it enhances or intensifies the natural salty taste of many processed foods. Although the additive is best known for its use in Chinese food, it is also incorporated into many other processed foods. MSG is made up of sodium and glutamate, or glutamic acid. Glutamic acid is an amino acid that is found naturally in the body and in high protein foods. The FDA classifies MSG as a "generally recognized as safe" additive. Because some people have an adverse reaction to it, the FDA requires all foods that contain MSG to indicate it as an ingredient on the label. In sensitive people, whether pregnant or not, MSG can trigger headaches, nausea, vomiting, sleep disturbances, and dizziness. More severe symptoms include breathing problems, chest pains, and increased blood pressure. Some studies in mice have shown possible birth defects and behavioral problems when MSG is consumed in large amounts, but no correlation has been established for humans. The FDA believes MSG is safe for the majority of the population to consume.

The bottom line is that if you are worried about ingesting MSG during pregnancy and how it may affect you and your baby, you should become aware of what foods contain it and limit your intake.

Olestra

Olean, also known as Olestra, is a noncaloric fat substitute that is made of a synthetic mixture of sugar and vegetable oil. Olestra was certified as safe by the FDA in 1996 and was approved for use in snack foods including potato chips, tortilla chips, and crackers. Some of these products include the Lay's WOW snacks, Doritos, and Pringles. Olestra basically passes through the body undigested. Because it is not absorbed, there is no danger in pregnant women of its reaching the fetus.

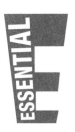

Remember that just because a food contributes no fat, it doesn't necessarily contain zero calories. Foods that contain Olestra will probably not harm you or your baby if eaten in moderation, but there are much better snack choices you can make.

However, there can be some negative effects from eating Olestra. It does interfere with the absorption of the fat-soluble vitamins A, D, E, and K. For that reason, the manufacturer is required to fortify Olestra products with those vitamins. The product also causes mild gastrointestinal discomfort such as diarrhea, gas, abdominal cramping, and greasy stools. The FDA initially required that Olestra products be labeled with a warning of the artificial fat's gastrointestinal affects. Recently, the FDA dropped the requirement because the effects are only mild for most people.

During pregnancy, you probably already deal with plenty of gastrointestinal discomforts. There is no need to compound these problems with foods that contain Olestra. In addition, they provide no real nutritional value. This is a time when you need foods that contain loads of nutrition. There are much better choices when it comes to snacks. Don't get yourself into the habit of snacking on chips, whether they contain fat or not. Instead, get in the habit of snacking on fruits, vegetables, yogurt, and other healthier foods.

Artificial Sweeteners

Artificial, or nonnutritive, sweeteners are added to all types of foods including gum, candy, sweets, soft drinks, and even to some over-the-counter medications. If you are trying to avoid these sweeteners or limit your consumption, read labels closely. Artificial sweeteners that are classified as "generally recognized as safe" are acceptable to use during pregnancy in moderation. However, the main health issue behind the use of artificial sweeteners is that they might encourage you to opt out of more nutritious foods. For example, if you drink gallons of diet soft drinks, you may not be drinking other more nutritious beverages such as water, milk, and juice that can be more beneficial. The other concern is that foods with artificial sweeteners are usually lower in calories, and pregnancy is not the time to be eating very low-calorie foods. Artificial sweeteners can be useful to pregnant women who have diabetes.

Aspartame

Aspartame is an artificial sweetener that is found in popular products such as NutraSweet, Equal, and most diet soft drinks. This sweetener has not been shown to cause birth defects, and the FDA considers moderate use during pregnancy to be safe.

Aspartame is a concern for women with phenylketonuria (PKU), a rare genetic disorder. Aspartame contains phenylalanine, an amino acid that is toxic for people with PKU. Women with PKU cannot break down phenyl-alanine, which can cause high levels in the mother's blood and may affect the developing fetus. Women who have the PKU gene, but not the disease, can break down aspartame well enough to keep from causing harm to their babies. If you have PKU, you should not consume aspartame. All products that contain aspartame have a phenylalanine warning label.

Saccharin

With all of the artificial sweeteners now on the market today, saccharin is much less commonly used. Saccharin is an artificial sweetener that is found in products such as Sweet 'n Low and some diet soft drinks as well as some over-the-counter medications. Saccharin was recently removed from the government's list of possible carcinogens after years of research. However, saccharin still carries a warning label until the FDA or Congress removes it.

Saccharin can cross the placenta and enter the baby's bloodstream. Research has shown that a baby clears saccharin from the bloodstream more slowly than the mother does. Whether this causes harm to the fetus or not is still a controversial issue. Some doctors may ban saccharin from their patient's diets. Because of the controversial and unknown safety of saccharin and unborn babies, it is suggested that saccharin be ingested in moderation if at all during pregnancy. Although there has been no concrete evidence that this sweetener is harmful to you or your baby, it is important to weigh the facts, speak to your doctor, and make your own personal decision.

Acesulfame-K

Acesulfame-K is one of the newer artificial sweeteners on the mar-ket. Acesulfame-K is marketed under the name Sunette. Acesulfame-K has recently been used in the product Pepsi One, which also includes aspartame, as well as candy, baked goods, desserts, and tabletop sweeteners such as Sweet One. The use of acesulfame-K within FDA guidelines appears safe for use during pregnancy.

Sucralose

Sucralose is one of the newest low-calorie sweeteners on the market and is the generic name for the product called Splenda. It was only approved by the FDA in 1998. This sweetener is actually made from sugar, but unlike sugar, it is not recognized as a carbohydrate during food digestion or absorption. The sweetener is not digested, absorbed, or metabolized for energy, so it does not affect blood sugar or insulin. Instead, sucralose basically passes through the body unchanged. Splenda can be found in many different products and is also packaged as a tabletop sweetener. Sucralose, or Splenda, is safe for pregnant women to consume, and as with other sweeteners it is best used in moderation.

The safety of FDA-approved nonnutritive sweeteners is expressed in terms of acceptable daily intake (ADI). This measure reflects the estimated amount per kilogram of body weight that a person can safely consume every day over a lifetime without health risk.

Sweetener	Acceptable Daily Intake*
Aspartame	50 mg/kilogram body weight
Saccharin	5 mg/kilogram body weight
Acesulfame K	15 mg/ kilogram body weight
Sucralose	0 to 15 mg/ kilogram body weight

*Weight in pounds divided by 2.2 will equal kilograms of body weight.

Something Fishy

Fish and seafood can be a valuable source of nutrition. Fish contains protein, omega-3 fatty acids, vitamin D, and other essential nutrients that make it an exceptionally healthy food for pregnant mothers and developing babies. However, some fish can contain harmful levels of methylmercury, a toxic mercury compound. Mercury occurs naturally in the environment and is often released into the air through industrial pollution. From the air, mercury can fall and accumulate in steams, lakes, and oceans where fish is caught for consumption. Bacteria in the water can cause chemical changes that transform mercury into the toxic form of methylmercury. Fish in these bodies of water absorb methylmercury as they feed on organisms within the water.

Harmful Effects

If consumed regularly by women who can become pregnant, women who are pregnant or nursing, or by a young child, methylmercury can harm a developing brain and nervous system. Just about all types of fish contain trace amounts of methylmercury, which is not harmful to most humans. However, larger fish that feed on other fish accumulate the highest levels of methylmercury. These types of fish pose the greatest risks to people that consume them on a regular basis. Pregnant women as well as women who are trying to conceive, nursing mothers, and young children are advised to also avoid these types of fish in large amounts. Women can avoid any risks associated with methylmercury and still get some of the important health benefits of fish by following the guidelines described in the following section.

Fish Guidelines

Any risk comes from a buildup of mercury in the body and not from a single meal. The Food and Drug Administration (FDA) and Environmental Protection Agency (EPA) have released specific advice concerning fish bought from stores and restaurants, which includes ocean and coastal fish as well as other types of commercial fish. If you follow the advice presented by the FDA and EPA, you can gain the positive benefits of eating fish while still avoiding any developmental problems to your baby due to the mercury content of fish. The FDA and EPA advise women who are pregnant or could become pregnant, nursing mothers, and young children not eat shark, swordfish, king mackerel, or tilefish because these fish contain higher unsafe levels of methylmercury.

Levels of methylmercury in other fish can vary. As a result, these agencies also advise that women who can become pregnant, women who are pregnant, and nursing mothers eat up to 12 ounces (2 average meals) a week of cooked fish or shellfish that are lower in mercury. Five of the most common fish that are low in mercury include shrimp, canned light tuna, salmon, pollock, and catfish. They also advise eating a variety of fish and shellfish and not eating the same type of fish or shellfish more than once per week.

If the fish is caught by family and friends in local lakes, rivers, and coastal areas, you should check local advisories about the safety of the type of fish caught. If no information or advice is available, you are advised to eat up to 6 ounces (one average meal) per week of the fish that was caught in local waters but don't eat any other fish during that same week. Follow these same guidelines for young children but with smaller portions. These guidelines are important when it comes to keeping the total level of methylmercury, contributed by all fish, to low levels in the body. It is smart to keep abreast of guidelines concerning the consumption of fish during pregnancy. Many organizations are trying to enforce stricter guidelines than are currently being recommended by the FDA and EPA. Check out the EPA Web site, at *www.epa.gov* and the FDA Web site at *www.fda.gov* for the latest advisories.

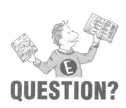

QUESTION?

Can I eat tuna salad while pregnant?
Guidelines released in March 2004 state that albacore tuna ("white tuna") as well as tuna steaks have higher mercury levels than canned light tuna. When you are choosing your two meals of fish and/or shellfish for the week, you can eat up to 6 ounces (one average meal) of albacore tuna per week. Even if you choose to use the canned light tuna, it is best to eat only one average meal of the tuna and choose another meal from another type of fish since the new advisory also suggests eating a variety of fish every week.

Sure About Soy?

Although soy can be a healthy alternative to animal foods, recent controversy questions its safety during pregnancy. Recent studies done on animals found that certain soy components consumed during pregnancy may adversely affect the sexual development of male offspring. Even though no effects have been observed in Asia, where soy is a major part of the diet, the studies have sparked concern and warrant further studies. Other concerns have been the plant-based hormones in soy that mimic estrogen. Research data is far from conclusive on these issues. In the meantime, it is best to remember the rule of thumb, which is moderation. If you are vegetarian, do not rely solely on soy for your main source of protein but choose other foods for variety. Also, it is best to consume soy in the form of whole soy foods rather than from dietary supplements containing soy in the form of pills and powders.

Drugs to Take and to Avoid

Some pills you pop, whether prescription or over-the-counter, may have dire consequences for your developing baby. Never assume anything is safe to take unless you speak to your doctor first. Many medications have not been studied extensively enough in pregnant women to determine whether they cause harm to the fetus. Therefore, it is vital to speak with your doctor before taking any type of medication. Taking some type of medication during pregnancy is not uncommon. The American Academy of Family Physicians estimate that more than 80 percent of pregnant women take over-the-counter or prescription drugs during pregnancy.

Prescription Medications

There is much controversy and plenty of gray area when it comes to the safety of prescription medications and pregnancy. There is no definitive answer on whether many medications are safe to use during pregnancy or not. Many do not have extensive, long-term studies that can give us clear-cut answers. The reality is that women can get sick during pregnancy, and many enter pregnancy with chronic conditions that require treatment with prescription medications.

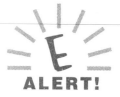

ALERT!

If you plan to get pregnant or become pregnant and are taking prescription medications, do not stop taking them without speaking with your doctor first. Many medications cannot be stopped abruptly without adverse effects and must be discontinued gradually.

Withholding medication during pregnancy is not always the answer, and sometimes there is more of a health risk to leaving a condition untreated. Medication use during pregnancy is common, and the number of a woman's prescriptions tends to rise with her age. The best that doctors can do is use the safest drug and safest dose possible so that all patients, including pregnant women, can receive the treatment they need.

It is absolutely vital that you speak with your doctor about all prescription medications you may be taking before you begin trying to conceive. Some medications that your doctor prescribed before you became pregnant may not be safe once you become pregnant. Your doctor can tell you what is safe and not safe to take and can make substitutions if necessary. Never take any prescription medication during pregnancy without speaking with your doctor first. If your doctor has prescribed a medication or deemed one safe to take, it is important to take the medication exactly as your doctor prescribes.

The FDA Ranking System

The FDA evaluates all available research studies that test the safety and efficacy of new drugs. Drugs are first tested on animals to determine their initial level of safety. Once they are deemed sufficiently safe, the drug is then tested on humans. These are controlled studies, in which one group takes the actual drug and another (the control group) takes a placebo. The problem with drugs and pregnancy is that due to the possible harm to the mother and fetus, they cannot be tested on pregnant women. Additionally, some drugs that are considered safe to take early in the first trimester may turn out to be harmful during the last trimester of pregnancy as the mother's body goes through physiological changes.

Some drugs are given an unclear safety rating when they are first made available, but they later receive a safe rating because many pregnant women used the drug during pregnancy with no harmful effects. To deal with this rating dilemma, the FDA created a rating system that assigns a safety category of A, B, C, D, or X to all over-the-counter and prescription drugs. These categories represent essential information about a drug's safety during pregnancy. This rating is required on the label of all drugs. Although the rating system has been under some scrutiny, it helps pregnant women and doctors to make important decisions about which drugs may be safe and what may not be safe to take.

The following is the ranking system of the FDA:

- **Category A**—Controlled studies have shown no risk. Adequate, well-controlled studies in pregnant women have failed to demonstrate a risk to the fetus in any trimester of pregnancy. Unfortunately, very few drugs fall into this category. Prenatal vitamins have a category A rating.
- **Category B**—Animal studies revealed no evidence of harm to the fetus; however, there are no adequate and well-controlled studies in pregnant women. Also in category B are drugs that have been shown to have an adverse effect in animal studies, but adequate and well-controlled studies in pregnant women have failed to demonstrate risk to the fetus.
- **Category C**—Risks cannot be ruled out. Adequate, well-controlled human studies are lacking, and animal studies have shown a risk to the fetus or are lacking as well. A category C implies that the drug may or may not be safe to take.
- **Category D**—Positive evidence of risk exists. Studies in humans, both controlled or observational (noncontrolled) studies, resulted in harm to the fetus. Nevertheless, potential benefits from the use of the drug may outweigh the potential risk. For example, the drug may be acceptable if needed in a life-threatening situation or serious disease for which safer drugs cannot be used or are ineffective (such as cancer treatment).
- **Category X**—The drug is contraindicated in pregnancy. Studies prove that the drug should never be used in any stage of pregnancy. Tests

demonstrate positive evidence of fetal abnormalities or risks, which clearly outweigh any possible benefit to the patient.

The bottom line is that all decisions regarding drug treatment during pregnancy should be made and monitored by your doctor.

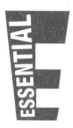

The FDA continually monitors the safety of drugs during pregnancy. Drug manufacturers are required to do their part by collecting feedback from pregnant women who are taking their drugs and to report their findings to the FDA.

Over-the-Counter Medications

In addition to prescription medications, over-the-counter medications can become a concern during pregnancy. Just because you can buy a product over the counter doesn't necessarily mean it is safe for you to take during pregnancy. Many over-the-counter products can be used safely during pregnancy under your doctor's supervision, but many can also be unsafe. Extensive testing is required for any drug before it can be labeled safe for use during pregnancy. The FDA ranking system categorizes all drugs.

Comprehensive, evidence-based guidelines for determining the safety of over-the-counter medications during pregnancy are not yet available. Ideally, any woman taking medication during pregnancy would be under the supervision of her doctor. Over-the-counter medications should not be used unless the benefits clearly outweigh the risks. Take the best care of yourself by seeking prenatal care, eating a healthy diet, and being physically active to decrease your chances of becoming ill or developing such problems as constipation. Seek alternative methods of relieving headaches, pains, and other problems before taking an over-the-counter medication.

Pain Relievers

Since 1984, all over-the-counter drug products have carried this warning: "As with any other drug, if you are pregnant or nursing, seek the advice of a health professional before using this product." In July 1990, the FDA issued an additional regulation requiring all oral and rectal nonprescription aspirin and drugs that contain aspirin to include this additional warning: "It is especially important not to use aspirin during the last three months of pregnancy unless specifically directed to do so by a doctor because it may cause problems in the unborn child or complications during delivery."

Aspirin is among one of the popular pain relievers. It is used for problems such as headaches, aches, pains, arthritis, and fevers. However, aspirin should not be taken during pregnancy unless specifically prescribed by your doctor. Aspirin may cause problems in the developing baby and complications during delivery and is classified as a category D in all three trimesters. Over-the-counter nonsteroidal anti-inflammatory drugs such as ibuprofen (Advil or Motrin), ketoprofen (Orudis), and naproxen (Aleve) also carry a warning that they should be used with caution in the first and second trimester and avoided during the third trimester. Acetaminophen (Tylenol), a category B during the entire course of pregnancy, is the pain reliever of choice recommended by most doctors.

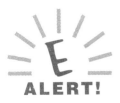

ALERT!

Just as important as what to take is how much to take. Always follow directions on the bottle or take as prescribed by your doctor. If an over-the-counter medication doesn't seem to do the trick, don't take more than directed without first speaking with your doctor. Only take over-the-counter medications as needed. If you have a headache, try lying down in a quiet place to see if you can relieve your headache before taking medication.

Decongestants, Expectorants, and Nonselective Antihistamines

Chlorpheniramine (Chlor-Trimeton), which falls in category B, is the antihistamine of choice for pregnant women. Also categorized as B is diphenhydramine (Benadryl), but it is suggested that you avoid this medication in your first trimester because it is known to cross the placenta. Clemastine fumarate (Tavist) has an unknown safety profile, even though it is classified as B. Pseudoephedrine hydrochloride (Novafed or Sudafed) is the oral decongestant of choice although oral decongestants should not be used unless absolutely necessary.

Topical nasal decongestants, such as oxymetazoline HCL (Afrin), can be recommended safely during pregnancy. Generally, patients should restrict their use to two to three sprays in each nostril twice a day for no more than three consecutive days. The cough suppressant Dextromethorphan hydrobromide (Benylin DM) appears to be safe during pregnancy. The expectorant Guaifenesin (Humibid L.A.) may be unsafe during the first trimester of pregnancy. Topical rubs such as Vicks Vapo Rub are safe during pregnancy.

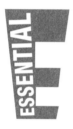

Some cold medicines contain alcohol, so you should use these sparingly if at all. Many cold medicines also contain pain relievers that may not be recommended, so read labels and ask your doctor before taking them.

Antidiarrheal, Constipation, and Laxative Medications

Kaolin and pectin (Kaopectate) is the antidiarrheal medication of choice for pregnant women because it does not cross the placenta. Pepto Bismol is not recommended because it can cross the placenta. Atropine/ diphenoxylate (Lomotil) is also not recommended due to questionable animal studies. Imodium is probably safe, but it is not recommended during the first trimester.

Bulking agents to help relieve constipation, such as Metamucil and Citrucel, are safe to use. To help relieve constipation, dietary intake, fluids, and regular exercise should be considered as the first course of treatment. If medication is needed, psyllium and bisacodyl (Dulcolax) are both considered safe during pregnancy. Laxatives and stool-softeners that are safe to use include Colace, Dulcolax, and Milk of Magnesia. Hemorrhoid creams safe to use include Tucks, Preparation H, and Anusol.

Indigestion, Gas, and Upset-Stomach Medications

Several forms of antacids are available over the counter, including preparations that contain alginic acid, aluminum, magnesium, and calcium. All of these are generally regarded as safe to take during pregnancy. Antacids for acid indigestion or heartburn that are safe to take include Tums, Rolaids, Mylanta, and Maalox. For gas problems, Gas-X, Mylanta Gas, Mylicon, and Phazyme are considered safe. Histamine H2-receptor blockers are effective in treating symptoms of heartburn and gastroesophageal reflux disease in pregnancy, but most cross the placenta. Their use is not recommended unless lifestyle change and antacids are ineffective in controlling the symptoms. Tagamet and Zantac are generally recommended only after antacids are tried first. Axid is not recommended due to questionable animal studies, and Pepcid is probably safe but more data is needed.

Herbal and All-Natural Supplements

There are hundreds of herbal and botanical supplements on the market today. Many pregnant women who wouldn't consider taking over-the-counter medications feel that herbal and botanical products are "natural" or "organic" and therefore safe. Never assume that just because a supplement is labeled "natural" or "organic" and is sold over the counter that it is safe to take during pregnancy. Little is known about the effects of herbal, botanical, and dietary supplements on a growing fetus and whether they are safe to use during pregnancy.

The dangers of herbal supplements are many. Supplements do not have to undergo the rigorous and extensive testing required by the FDA for prescription and over-the-counter medications. There are no required standards for the amounts of active ingredients contained in herbal supplements—these can vary wildly among different brands. Some supplements can also interact with medications and reduce their effectiveness.

Warnings

Common remedies used for nausea and vomiting such as red raspberry, wild yam, and homeopathic treatments have not been scientifically studied.

Some are known to be harmful. These include comfrey, which may cause liver damage; blue cohosh, which may cause heart defects; and pennyroyal, which could cause spontaneous abortions.

Keep in mind that herbal teas may also contain substances that may not be safe. If you do use herbal teas, don't drink more than a few cups per day, and be sure your doctor knows you are drinking the tea. Teas considered safe include blackberry, citrus peel, ginger, lemon balm, orange peel, and rose hip if they have been processed according to government safety standards. Don't assume these teas are caffeine-free, and always check the label to be sure they include no added substances.

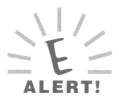

ALERT!

Although you should question all herbal and botanical supplements, a few popular herbs are suspected in particular of being harmful during pregnancy. These include aloe, chamomile, black cohosh, blue cohosh, devil's claw root, dong quai, ephedra, eucalyptus, fenugreek, feverfew, ginseng, guarana, hawthorne, juniper, licorice, St. John's Wort, and willow. Again, this is only a sampling of some herbal supplements that may not be safe; there are hundreds more on the market. You should check out each one, and speak to your doctor before taking any.

While some herbal ingredients have undergone extensive testing, the safety and effectiveness of many herbal supplements have not been demonstrated at all. To ensure safety, it is best to stay away from any herbal product during pregnancy unless you have permission from your doctor. Don't let herbs become a substitute for medical attention, especially during pregnancy when specific symptoms can be signs of other problems.

If you have bothersome symptoms and do not want to risk taking over-the-counter medications, do not take matters into your own hands by taking what you think is "natural." Instead, speak to your doctor. Also, be careful of taking the advice of others or the advice of people selling these supplements. These people don't always have your best interest at heart and don't always have all the facts.

Always check with your doctor before beginning to take an herbal supplement or continuing an herbal supplement that you were taking before becoming pregnant. To ensure the best outcome for you and your baby, always discuss any over-the-counter medication, prescription medication, dietary supplement, and/or herbal supplement with your doctor.

Meal Replacement Supplements

You can find all kinds of meal-replacement bars, drinks, and powders on the market today. Are they safe to use? This can be a tricky question. These products are probably safe unless they contain herbal products or other substances deemed unsafe during pregnancy. It is also possible for these products to contain high amounts of vitamins that could be toxic for pregnant women, such as vitamin A. Some may also be high in protein. Even though your protein needs are slightly increased, too much protein can put undue stress on your body. These products are not formulated for pregnant women, and you are best sticking with wholesome foods. If there is a product that you like and want to continue eating, consult with your doctor or a dietitian before making it part of your regular diet.

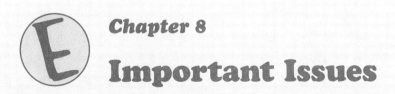

Chapter 8

Important Issues

If you are pregnant, you probably have a variety of concerns related to keeping your baby as safe as possible. You need to know how to deal with important issues and be aware of safety issues that exist. This chapter touches on some important issues that can be of special concern during pregnancy.

Dealing with Lactose Intolerance

Dealing with lactose intolerance during pregnancy can present a challenge. If you are lactose intolerant, you are not alone. It is estimated that between 30 and 50 million Americans suffer from lactose intolerance. Being lactose intolerant means that you have an intolerance to lactose, which is the sugar naturally found in milk and milk products. During digestion, an enzyme called lactase helps to break lactose down into smaller, more easily digested sugars. People who are lactose intolerant do not produce enough lactase to do the job properly. When lactose is left undigested, it can cause symptoms such as nausea, cramping, bloating, abdominal pain, gas, and diarrhea. Lactose intolerance can affect people in varying degrees. Some people may have more or more severe symptoms than others. Other people may be able to consume small amounts of milk and milk products with no symptoms.

Symptoms of Lactose Intolerance

Symptoms of lactose intolerance can be noticeable as soon as fifteen minutes after ingestion of lactose-containing foods, or they make take several hours to kick in. Lactose intolerance is not an all-or-nothing type of problem. It is a matter of degree and a matter of how much your body can tolerate. Women who are lactose intolerant before becoming pregnant can see an increase in symptoms or possibly a decrease during pregnancy.

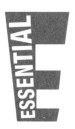

Being lactose intolerance does not mean you are allergic to milk and milk products. Allergies and intolerances are two completely different problems. A food allergy involves the body's immune system, but a food intolerance does not. A true milk allergy means you are allergic to a protein found in milk, such as casein. People who suffer from milk allergies can have severe allergic symptoms such as hives and breathing problems and must avoid all milk and milk products. Less than 2 percent of the adult population actually has true milk allergies.

If you experience symptoms during pregnancy and have never been lactose intolerant in the past, it could be that the symptoms are due to changes in your body during pregnancy. They could also be caused by another condition. If you were not lactose intolerant before your pregnancy, but you notice symptoms during pregnancy, do not diagnose yourself. Instead, speak with your doctor immediately concerning your symptoms. If you are severely lactose intolerant during pregnancy and cannot tolerate any milk or milk products, your doctor may need to prescribe additional nutrients, such as calcium.

Maintaining Calcium Levels

If you are pregnant and suffering from lactose intolerance, you must avoid or decrease your intake of milk and milk products. The concern here has to do with the essential nutrients that you may be missing. The main nutrients in milk and milk products that may be of concern include calcium and vitamin D.

Even though you may be lactose intolerant, there are steps you can take to help maintain your level of nutrients such as calcium. To help manage your lactose intolerance, it is important to experiment with varying amounts of milk and dairy products to see what you can tolerate. Start with small amounts, and gradually increase the portion size to determine your personal tolerance level. Some dairy products seem to be better tolerated than others. Yogurt, for example, has lactose that is already partially digested by the cultured bacteria it contains, so it may be easier for you to tolerate. Look for the National Yogurt Association's seal, "Live and Active Cultures," on yogurt cartons. Some buttermilk is also made with active cultures.

Always read food labels and ingredient lists for words that may indicate a product includes lactose, such as milk, dry milk solids, nonfat milk solids, buttermilk, lactose, malted milk, sour or sweet cream, margarine, milk chocolate, whey, whey protein concentrate, and cheese. If you still enjoy your cereal and milk at breakfast, try lactose-reduced or lactose-free milk and dairy products. If you choose lactose-free milk, ensure it contains calcium. You can also try calcium-fortified soy milk as an alternative, which is lactose free. Be aware that some baked and processed foods often contain some amount of lactose, so get in the habit of checking labels.

To help your system tolerate lactose-containing foods, eat them as part of a meal rather than alone. The mix of foods can help slow down the release of lactose into the digestive system, helping to make it easier to digest. Choose calcium-rich foods that are naturally lower in lactose, such as aged cheeses (Swiss, Colby, Parmesan, or Cheddar). As a quick tip, look for kosher foods that have the words "parev" or "parve" on the label. This means they are milk-free. Try consuming dairy products in smaller quantities at one sitting. Instead of drinking a whole glass of milk, split it up to ½ cup with lunch and ½ cup with dinner. You can also try special tablets and drops that you can add to regular milk that will help to break down the lactose before you drink it. Make sure to follow package directions. There are also lactase enzyme tablets that you can take before eating milk or milk products.

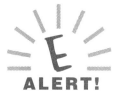

ALERT!

Do not diagnose yourself, and do not begin to take additional calcium and vitamin D without speaking to your doctor first. Neither of these nutrients should be taken in excess.

If you are lactose intolerant, it is important to add calcium-rich foods other than dairy products to your daily intake to ensure you get all you need. Include foods such as dark-green leafy vegetables, calcium-fortified products such as orange juice and cereal, soybeans, almonds, and canned sardines or salmon with bones. Also important are foods that are good sources of vitamin D, including canned salmon with bones, fortified cereals, eggs, and margarines.

What's up with Pica?

Pica is the name for a condition in which a person craves nonfood substances, such as dirt (geophagia), soap, laundry starch, ice, or chalk. The word "pica" actually comes from the Latin word for magpie, a bird known for eating just about anything. Pica is seen in young children and, less commonly, in pregnant women. Pica seems to occur more in African-American women and in those women who have a family or childhood history of pica. Most women have cravings while pregnant, but most crave food substances. Pica cravings are less common, but they do occur. Because pregnant women who practice pica risk the chance of being exposed to toxicants such as lead and other harmful substances, your doctor should be notified immediately if you experience these types of cravings. The most common substances related to pica cravings include dirt, clay, and laundry starch. Others include burnt matches, stones, charcoal, mothballs, ice, cornstarch, soap, sand, toothpaste, plaster, baking soda, paint chips, cigarette ashes, and coffee grounds.

Causes and Effects of Pica

The cause of pica is not really known. There is speculation that pica cravings occur as a result of the body's attempt to obtain vitamins and minerals that it is not getting from foods. The American Dietetic Association feels there is a possible connection between pica and iron deficiency. Still others suspect pica could be related to probable underlying physical or mental illnesses.

A pregnant woman who gives in to these unusual cravings and eats these nonfood substances can potentially harm herself and her developing fetus. These substances can interfere with the body's ability to absorb nutrients from healthy foods and can cause deficiencies. There is also a concern that the substances consumed may contain toxic or parasitic ingredients. These substances can cause all type of problems, such as bowel obstruction, constipation, and intestinal pain.

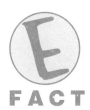

FACT

Ice consumption in large amounts is not toxic to your system, but there is some evidence that women who eat ice daily in amounts of ½ cup to 2 cups have lower levels of iron in the blood in the second and third trimesters.

What to Do About Pica Cravings

If you experience these abnormal cravings, the first thing to do is inform your doctor immediately. Gather as much information as possible about the specific risks associated with your specific craving. Do not be embarrassed to speak to your doctor about your unusual cravings! If you have been consuming any of these substances, you may need to be tested and/or monitored for toxic substances you have ingested.

Your doctor may monitor you for nutritional deficiencies. She also may assess your iron intake along with your intake of other vitamin and minerals through both supplements and healthy foods. Try to find substitutes for your cravings. Chew sugarless gum or suck on sugarless candy. Inform your spouse or a friend who can help act as support and keep you accountable.

Cold and Flu Season

Even if you have the best intentions and take optimal care of yourself, you may not be able to completely protect yourself from catching a cold or the flu virus while you are pregnant. Though you may decrease your chances, you are still vulnerable. Because of changes in your immune system during pregnancy, symptoms from colds and/or the flu can persist longer than normal. Pregnancy also increases the risk of complications from the flu and other viruses. Call your doctor immediately if you come down with any type of illness. Some viruses, such as those that cause chickenpox or Fifth disease, can be more dangerous if contracted during pregnancy. If you come in contact with anyone who is infected with these or any other contagious illness, contact your doctor immediately.

Protecting Yourself

Eating a healthy diet (one that includes all the food groups in proper amounts), drinking plenty of water, and exercising regularly can definitely decrease your chances of becoming sick while you are pregnant. However, you may need to take additional steps and be extra careful during the cold and flu season. Be careful of the contact you have with family or friends, including children, who may be sick. Wash your hands regularly to lessen the risk of coming in contact with virus germs, especially in public places. Make your visits to crowded places less frequent, as they can be a breeding ground for germs.

If you will be more than three months pregnant during the flu season, you should talk to your doctor about getting a flu shot. If you have medical problems such as diabetes that can increase your risk of complications from the flu, talk to your doctor about getting a flu shot, no matter what trimester you are in.

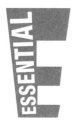

Because flu shots are actually made from inactivated viruses, many doctors consider the flu shot safe during all stages of pregnancy. However, since miscarriages most often occur in the first trimester of pregnancy, most doctors do not routinely administer flu shots during the first trimester to avoid any possible problems. There seems to be no harm to the baby if the vaccine is given while you are breastfeeding. Speak to your doctor before getting a flu shot.

Measures to Take

Classic flu symptoms such as fever, severe muscle aches, nasal congestion, upper respiratory symptoms, and gastrointestinal symptoms can be bothersome for anyone, but this is especially true for pregnant women. If you do catch a cold or the flu, the following measures will help you to deal more comfortably with your symptoms:

- Increase your fluid intake. Water is important, but beverages such as juice will provide extra fluids and nutrition at a time when you may have a decrease in appetite. Proper hydration can also help to thin out nasal congestion.
- Try to maintain your nutritional intake with small meals throughout the day. Stick to foods that are bland and easily digestible.
- Get plenty of rest.
- If you are having problems with nasal congestion, elevate your head when lying down to help enhance your breathing.

- Use a vaporizer or steam to help loosen congestion.
- Use warm compresses to help alleviate sinus pain caused by congestion.
- For a sore throat, try gargling with warm salt water.
- To ease achy muscles, take a warm bath.

Monitor your body temperature often, and call your doctor if it rises over 101°F. Don't take any over-the-counter medications until you speak with your doctor, especially if you are still in your first trimester.

If you are experiencing nausea, vomiting, and/or diarrhea (not associated with common morning sickness) contact your doctor, and make sure you are getting plenty of fluids. It is important to maintain your nutritional intake. A liquid diet, such as juice, water, tea, Jell-O, clear soups or broth, ice chips, Gatorade, and Popsicles during this time can be helpful. Once a clear liquid diet can be tolerated, other foods can be introduced slowly. Once your appetite begins to return, start slowly by introducing food such as milkshakes, toast, dry cereal, and crackers.

Food Safety Awareness

Although the food supply in the Unites States is one of the safest in the world, the way we store, prepare, and/or handle food after it leaves the grocery store can put us at risk for foodborne illness or food poisoning. Some foods can carry harmful bacteria and parasites that can make both you and your baby sick. Pregnant women are in the higher-risk category when it comes to contracting foodborne bacteria, such as salmonella, staphylococcus aureus, E. coli, clostridium perfringens, toxoplasma gondii, or listeria monocyotogenes. Some foodborne bacteria can be more harmful to the mother and baby than others.

Symptoms of Foodborne Illness

Symptoms of foodborne illnesses can develop as soon as thirty minutes or as much as three weeks after a contaminated food is eaten. Since symptoms can mimic those of the flu, it is important to know the differences. If you have flu-like symptoms but they don't go away within twenty-four to forty-eight hours, that could be a sign of something more serious, such as foodborne illness. If you vomit; have diarrhea more than two times per day; have bloody diarrhea; have a stiff neck with a severe headache and fever; or if your symptoms last for more than three days, you should call your doctor immediately. Foodborne illnesses can be serious, so don't take any chances. If you have any symptoms, see your doctor immediately so he can determine what is causing your discomfort. If your doctor suspects a foodborne illness, he can perform a blood antibody test for certain bacteria or parasites.

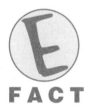

FACT

Toxoplasma gondii, or T. gondii, is a parasitic infection that can contaminate food. This parasite can result in toxoplasmosis, which usually causes mild to no symptoms for pregnant women but there is a 40 percent chance that it can be passed to the developing fetus. T. gondii can cause miscarriage, disability, and retardation. Toxoplasmosis is sometimes treated with antibiotics to reduce the severity of its effects. Most often, it is contracted from eating undercooked meat and poultry or unwashed fruits and vegetables, from contamination of cleaning a cat's litter box, or from handling contaminated soil.

Listeria Monocyotogenes

Listeria monocytogenes is a bacteria on some foods that can cause a serious infection, called listeriosis, in humans. Most people who eat listeria-contaminated foods do not get ill. However, pregnant women are twenty times more likely than other healthy adults to get listeriosis and become seriously ill. Listeriosis results in an estimated 2,500 serious illnesses and 500 deaths each year.

Pregnant women, older adults, and people with weakened immune systems are at higher risk for contracting listeriosis. This foodborne illness is one that can cause the most serious harm to a fetus, resulting in miscarriages, fetal death, severe illness, and even the death of a newborn. If a person has three telltale symptoms—stiff neck, severe headache, and fever—she may have listeria.

Foods to Avoid

Listeria monocytogenes can grow at refrigerator temperatures and can be found in ready-to-eat foods. Listeria can also contaminate other foods, and contaminated foods may not look, smell, or even taste any different than uncontaminated foods. Eat perishable foods that are precooked or ready-to-eat as soon as possible. Clean your refrigerator on a regular basis, and keep a thermometer in your refrigerator to make sure it stays at 40°F or below. These steps can help reduce your risk for listeriosis as well as other foodborne illnesses. Thorough cooking at the correct temperatures can kill the listeria bacteria.

Some foods have a greater likelihood of containing listeria monocytogenes and can put you are greater risk for other foodborne illnesses. Pregnant women should *completely avoid* the following foods:

- Hot dogs and luncheon meats, unless they are reheated until steaming hot (at least 165°F)
- Soft cheeses such as feta (goat cheese), Brie, Camembert, blue-veined cheeses such as Roquefort, and Mexican-style soft cheeses such as queso blanco fresco. It is acceptable to eat hard cheese such as Cheddar; semi-soft cheese such as mozzarella; pasteurized processed cheese such as slices and spreads; cream cheeses; and cottage cheese
- Pâtés and/or meat spreads. It is acceptable to eat canned or shelf-stable pâtés and meat spreads
- Refrigerated smoked seafood, unless contained in a cooked dish such as a casserole
- Raw (unpasteurized) milk or foods that contain unpasteurized milk. Foods and beverages state "pasteurized" on the label
- Unpasteurized juices and ciders
- Raw sprouts
- Dishes including raw or undercooked eggs including eggnog, cake batter, raw cookie dough, some Caesar salad dressings, and hollandaise sauce. Check for ingredients on food labels
- Raw or undercooked shellfish or seafood, including sushi
- Undercooked meats, poultry, and eggs

Steps to Keep Food Safe

Since you cannot always tell whether a food is contaminated, it is vital to take important steps to keep all of your food safe from harmful bacteria. To decrease your risk of contracting a foodborne illness, always wash your hands with hot, soapy water before and after handling foods. In addition, wash cutting boards, other work surfaces, and utensils with soap and hot water after contact with raw meat, poultry, or fish. In fact, it is best to use separate cutting boards, plates, storage containers, and utensils for raw meat and other foods. Thoroughly cooking all meat, poultry, and seafood can greatly help decrease the risk of contracting a foodborne illness. To help prevent listeria, reheat all meats purchased at the deli counter, including cured meats like salami, before eating them. Keep your raw foods separate from cooked or ready-to-eat foods so they don't contaminate them. Change sponges, dishcloths, and dishrags frequently. Always wash fruits and vegetables thoroughly with warm water before eating, and remove surface dirt with a scrub brush. Refrigerate all of your leftovers promptly, and stay away from cooked food that has been out of the refrigerator for more than two hours. Use a thermometer to make sure that the temperature in your refrigerator is 40°F or below and that the freezer is 0°F or below to slow the growth of bacteria. The danger zone for foods is between 40 and 140°F. Thawing meats and seafood can be a breeding ground for bacteria if they are not defrosted properly. The safest way to thaw frozen meats or seafood is in the refrigerator. Pay attention to labels on products that must be refrigerated or that have a "use by" date. Avoid dented or swollen cans, cracked jars, and loose lids that can contain bacteria. The best rule of thumb is "When in doubt, throw it out!"

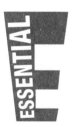

When cooking meats, use a meat thermometer to ensure meats are cooked thoroughly. Make sure ground meat products are cooked to at least 160°F. Roasts and steaks should be cooked to at least 145°F for medium rare and 170°F for well done. Pork should be cooked to at least 160°F. Poultry should be cooked to at least 180°F for whole chickens, turkeys, and dark meat and to 170°F for white-meat breasts and roasts.

New information and guidelines on food safety are frequently available. Since pregnancy puts you and your baby at higher risk for food-borne illnesses, it is prudent advice for you to keep up with the most current information. Check out the U.S. government's food safety Web site at *www.foodsafety.gov.*

Tips to Travel By

There is a good chance you will want or need to travel at some point in your pregnancy. Traveling by any means, including car and plane, can be safe if thoughtfully planned out. Your second trimester is usually the safest time to travel in terms of your physical comfort and the risk of miscarriage or labor. For most women, morning sickness has subsided by this time. The best travel advice is that you should plan ahead and consult with your doctor before making any travel arrangements.

The American College of Obstetrics and Gynecology advises that the safest time for pregnant women to travel is during the second trimester (eighteen to twenty-four weeks). That is the point at which you will most likely feel your best, and it is when the danger of spontaneous abortion or premature labor is least. Pregnant women can also fly safely to up to thirty-six weeks gestation.

Nutritional Advice

When traveling, especially by airplane, women need to concentrate on staying well hydrated. Water is the best thing you can drink, followed by fruit juices. If you are traveling internationally, stick to bottled water. Avoid water in its hidden forms, such as in ice, prepared salads, and vegetables that may be washed in water. The vomiting and diarrhea that can sometimes be caused by contaminated water can quickly lead to dehydration. Most medications that are normally given in this situation are not safe during pregnancy.

Dehydration can also be a particular problem when you are flying or traveling to a humid, hot, or high-altitude area. To make sure you are well hydrated, look for signs of dehydration such as thirst, dark yellow urine (though this can also occur if you are taking prenatal vitamins), muscle cramping, or a dry mouth and nose. More serious symptoms include dizziness, weakness, and/or lethargy. Stay away from caffeinated beverages at this time, as they can act as a diuretic. If you are in excessively hot weather, you may want to grab a sports drink that includes electrolytes.

When flying, drink water throughout your flight to combat the dry cabin air. If traveling by car or bus, take healthy snacks and bottles of water that will last throughout your trip. Try to stop frequently, and get out to stretch your legs. Sitting for long periods of time can cause you to experience leg cramps, discomfort, and fatigue, especially in the last trimester. Don't forget to take your prenatal vitamins with you, and continue to stick to your healthy pregnancy diet—no matter where you travel!

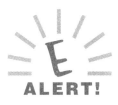

ALERT!

High altitudes of greater than 2,500 meters or 8,200 feet should be avoided in late or high-risk pregnancies. Pregnant women who are traveling to a higher-altitude area should postpone physical activity until they become acclimated.

International Travel

If you are planning to travel internationally, be sure that the country has appropriate facilities and doctors to care for pregnant women. Plan ahead; some countries may require immunizations that are not safe to receive during pregnancy. In foreign countries be careful to avoid foods that are raw or undercooked as well as unpasteurized foods, such as milk and cheese. It may be common practice in other countries to eat foods in different preparations than in the United States. Many foreign countries do not have as safe a food supply as the United States.

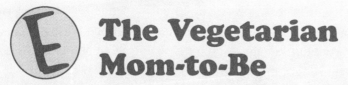

Chapter 9

The Vegetarian Mom-to-Be

Being pregnant does not mean you have to give up your vegetarian lifestyle. However, just as with any other eating style, if you are following a vegetarian diet during pregnancy, you must ensure that you get well-balanced and varied meals. Although the typical vegetarian diet is very low in saturated fat and cholesterol, not all diets are low in calories, total fat, or sugar. Some can also be lacking in other essential vitamins and minerals unless they are properly planned.

What Type Are You?

Before discussing the pros and cons of following a vegetarian diet during pregnancy, it is necessary to be aware that there are difference types of vegetarian diets. People turn to vegetarian diets for all kinds of reasons, including religious, ethical, environmental, and personal health concerns. For some, vegetarianism is simply a way of eating while for others it is a way of life. There are different types of vegetarian eating styles, and each one differs as to what nutrients may be missing and what adjustments might be necessary to ensure optimal nutritional intake during pregnancy.

Vegetarianism is a type of eating style that is a matter of personal choice. Some people choose to avoid all animal products, while others may choose to consume some animal foods such as eggs and/or dairy products (lacto-ovo vegetarian). Only a small percentage of vegetarians are strict vegetarians, or vegans, who avoid all animal products. The majority of vegetarians in the United States fit into the lacto-ovo vegetarian category.

Vegetarians are classified into several different categories, as follows:

- **Vegan or strict vegetarian**—Absolutely no animal foods, including meat, fish, poultry, eggs, milk, or other dairy products. Also, no foods made with any type of animal product, such as refried beans made with lard or baked goods made with eggs.
- **Lacto vegetarian**—Dairy foods permitted, but no other animal foods including eggs and meat (meat, poultry, fish, and seafood.)
- **Lacto-ovo vegetarian**—Dairy foods and eggs permitted, but no other animal foods, including meats (meat, poultry, fish, and seafood).
- **Semi-vegetarian**—A mostly vegetarian diet (lacto-ovo-vegetarian), but meat, poultry, or fish permitted occasionally.

Is a Vegetarian Diet Safe During Pregnancy?

With careful planning, a vegetarian diet, no matter what the type, can be healthy and safe during pregnancy. It is essential to assess your intake of certain nutrients that are especially important during pregnancy. These nutrients include vitamin B_{12}, calcium, vitamin D, iron, zinc, and protein.

If you follow a lacto-ovo or a lacto vegetarian diet, meaning you include dairy or dairy and eggs in your eating plan, you have fewer nutritional hurdles to get over. If you are vegan, you have to be much more vigilant about consuming all of the essential nutrients you need for a healthy pregnancy. That includes making sure that you consume enough calories recommended for pregnancy. Vegetarians, especially vegans, should keep tabs on their weight gain during pregnancy.

The Benefits

Vegetarian diets can be very healthy if designed correctly. A healthy, well-planned vegetarian diet usually contains more fiber. It is also lower in total fat, especially saturated fat and dietary cholesterol, which can help lower the risk for diseases such as heart disease, stroke, and some cancers. In addition, LDL blood cholesterol (the "bad" cholesterol) levels are generally lower in vegetarians, which can decrease the incidence of death from heart disease. Vegetarians tend to have a lower incidence of hypertension, Type 2 diabetes, obesity, and some forms of cancers such as lung and colon, than people who eat meat. Vegetarian diets that are high in fruits, vegetables, and whole grains also tend to be higher in folic acid, antioxidants such as vitamins C and E, carotenoids, and phytochemicals. All these benefits give this eating style an extra disease-fighting punch. However, the key to being at a lower risk for these health problems is following a properly balanced vegetarian diet.

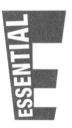

Keep in mind that not all vegetarian protein sources are low in fat. Popular protein sources, such as nuts and seeds, can be high in fat. These contain unsaturated (or healthy) fats, but small amounts can pack in lots of calories.

The Pitfalls

It is important to keep in mind that being a vegetarian does not guarantee that you are eating a healthy diet. A poorly planned vegetarian diet can cause some nutritional deficiencies. It can also be high in fat, cholesterol, and calories and low in fiber. Some vegetarians may have a high saturated-fat intake from consuming too many eggs, cream, butter, whole-milk products, and cheese. Vegetarians may get into the rut of eating too many low-fiber starches without including enough of the other food groups, such as plant-based proteins, fruits, vegetables, whole grains, and dairy foods (if included in their eating style).

Despite some of the pitfalls of a vegetarian diet, you can still reap the benefits of a vegetarian lifestyle as long as you plan your meals correctly and you eat higher fat, higher sugar foods in moderation.

A Balanced Pregnancy Diet

A healthy vegetarian pregnancy diet must be balanced. In other words, it must contain all of the nutrients essential to good health and a healthy pregnancy. It may take a little work, but keep in mind that knowledge is power. The more you know about the foods you eat, the more nutritious your diet can become. The nutritional adequacy of a vegetarian diet depends more on the overall food choices made over several days than what you consume at each meal.

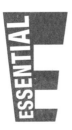

During breastfeeding, you need more calories than you do while pregnant. Vegetarian women who are breastfeeding also need to make sure they are consuming plenty of vitamin B_{12} sources because intake can affect levels in breast milk. While you are on prenatal vitamins, you should get all of the nutrients you need. After delivery, your doctor will most likely take you off your prenatal vitamins. Talk to your doctor or a dietitian about starting a multivitamin/mineral supplement that will ensure optimal nutritional intake.

The Vegetarian Food Guide Pyramid

The Vegetarian Food Guide Pyramid is very similar to the regular Food Guide Pyramid. The vegetarian version provides recommended guidelines for the vegetarian population. The lacto-ovo vegetarian diet can be modified to meet the guidelines of the Food Guide Pyramid with only a few modifications. If you consume eggs and/or dairy products, choose lower-fat or nonfat products to limit the amount of saturated fat and cholesterol you consume each day.

The following list describes the minimum number of servings you should consume from each food group during pregnancy:

- *Use fats, oils, and sweets sparingly.* This includes candy, butter, margarine, salad dressing, and cooking oil.
- *Eat 3–4 servings from the milk, yogurt, and cheese group.* Examples of single servings from this group include one cup of milk or yogurt or 1.5 ounces of cheese. Vegetarians who choose not to eat milk, yogurt, or cheese should select other food sources rich in calcium, such as calcium-fortified juice, cereal, dark-green leafy vegetables, and soy milk.
- *Eat 2 servings (6–7 ounces each) from the dry beans, nuts, seeds, eggs, and meat substitutes group.* Examples of a single serving from this food group include one cup of soy milk, ½ cup of cooked dry beans or peas, one egg or two egg whites, 1/3 cup of nuts or seeds, or 2 tablespoons peanut butter. Shoot to eat at least 3–4 servings of cooked dried beans weekly. They are a good choice because they are full of zinc, iron, protein, and fiber.
- *Eat 4 servings from the vegetable group.* Examples of a single serving from this group include ½ cup of cooked or chopped raw vegetables or 1 cup of raw leafy vegetables. Choose dark-green leafy vegetables often for higher calcium intake.
- *Eat 3 servings from the fruit group.* Examples of a single serving from this group include ¾ cup of juice, ¼ cup of dried fruit, ½ cup of chopped raw fruit, ½ cup of canned fruit, or a medium-size piece of fruit, such as banana, apple, or orange.
- *Eat 9 servings from the bread, cereal, rice, and pasta group.* Examples of a single serving from this group include one slice of bread, 1 ounce of ready-to-eat cereal, ½ cup of cooked cereal, ½ cup of cooked brown rice, pasta, or other grains, or half a bagel. Choose whole-wheat and whole-grain breads and pastas more often, as well as fortified and enriched products.

Vegetarian Meal Planning Tips

The key to a vegetarian diet is making the right choices and eating a variety of foods. It never hurts to take an overall look at your diet to make sure it is well balanced, nutritious, and in line with your new pregnancy needs. There are all kinds of vegetarian foods out there that you may have never thought of trying. Here are a few suggestions to get you started:

- Explore new foods at your grocery store. Instead of going with the same old foods, try new grains (such as barley, bulgur, couscous, kasha, and quinoa), vegetables, and/or legumes each week.
- Try different meat-free or soy products from the selection located in the freezer section or the health section. Soy can boost the protein, calcium, and iron content of almost any meal.
- Add different types of legumes or dried beans to casseroles, stews, soups, salads, and chili for a protein, iron, zinc, and fiber boost to your meal.
- Prepare some of your favorite dishes with a soy substitute, such as using textured vegetable protein in Sloppy Joes or spaghetti sauce or adding cubed tofu to a stir-fry along with your favorite vegetables.
- Next time you grill out, try a marinated portabella mushroom or veggie burger marinated in teriyaki sauce or your favorite marinade.
- Buy a vegetarian cookbook, or search out meatless recipes on the Internet for new ideas. The Web sites *www.vegweb.com*, *www.fatfree.com*, and *www.vegkitchen.com* should get you started.
- When looking for a place to dine out, suggest Chinese, Vietnamese, Thai, or Italian. You can always find plenty of vegetarian entrees on these menus.

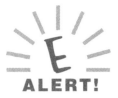

If you are a vegan, you will have a tougher time making sure you receive all the essential nutrients you need during pregnancy. You will need to make more modifications to the Food Guide Pyramid. Seek the guidance of a dietitian who can make sure you are planning your diet correctly.

Special Vitamin and Mineral Considerations

If you are not careful, eliminating animal foods from your diet can cause a shortfall of several nutrients in an otherwise healthy eating plan. Nutrients that should be given special attention include calcium, vitamin D, iron, vitamin B_{12}, and zinc. You should notify your doctor of your vegetarian eating style so that she is aware of your nutrient intake and can prescribe supplements you might need. In addition, careful meal planning and good choices can ensure the intake of all these essential nutrients each day. Keep in mind that you should never take additional supplements without first speaking to your doctor. It is possible to overdo a good thing! If you have questions about how you can combine foods to incorporate essential vitamins and minerals, speak to a registered dietitian.

Calcium

Calcium is vital for strong bones and teeth for both the baby and the mother. Pregnant women need 1,000 mg per day. For vegetarian moms who consume dairy products (at least three servings of dairy foods each day), consuming enough calcium should not be a problem. For vegans, however, calcium intake can be a concern. However, calcium can be found in both plant and animal foods.

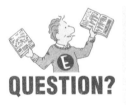

QUESTION?

Is it OK to take a calcium supplement if I don't eat dairy foods?
If you can't get enough calcium from the foods you choose, a supplement can be a good idea. The rule of thumb should always be food before supplements, though. First, include calcium-containing foods in your diet as much as possible, and then supplement on top of that. Never let a supplement take the place of an entire food group or nutrient such as calcium.

Though it may take a bit more planning, as a pregnant vegan you can definitely find foods that fit your eating style and contain enough calcium to help you meet your daily needs. Some of these foods include tofu processed with calcium; calcium-fortified beverages such as orange juice and soy milk; calcium-fortified breakfast cereals; broccoli; seeds, such as sunflower and sesame; tahini; nuts such as almonds; soy beans; legumes; some greens, such as kale, mustard greens, and collards; bok choy; okra; dried figs; almond butter; and some dark-green leafy vegetables.

Vitamin D

Vitamin D is essential to help the body absorb calcium and phosphorus and then depositing them into teeth and bones. Your body can also make vitamin D when your skin is exposed to sunlight. With the exception of milk, very few foods are naturally high in vitamin D. If you are a vegetarian who drinks milk, vitamin D should not be a concern if you consume the recommended number of servings. However, if you are a vegan, you need to be careful that you get enough vitamin D in your diet. The best way for vegans to get vitamin D is from fortified foods. Check the nutrition facts panel on the labels of foods fortified with vitamin D, such as breakfast cereals, soy beverages, and some calcium-fortified juices. Your prenatal vitamin should also ensure that you are receiving the amount of vitamin D you need daily for a healthy pregnancy. The requirement for pregnant women is 5 mcg per day.

Iron

Regardless of whether you are a vegetarian, it is likely that you don't get enough iron. This nutrient is often lacking in women's diets. As a result, during pregnancy, women are often prescribed a prenatal vitamin and mineral supplement that includes iron to meet their increased needs and to prevent iron-deficiency anemia. As a pregnant vegetarian, it can be difficult to get enough absorbable iron to meet your daily needs.

Some plant foods do contain iron. Called nonheme iron, it is not absorbed as well as the iron found in animal foods, or heme iron. The challenge for vegetarians is to improve the absorption of nonheme iron foods. You can start by consuming iron-rich plant sources every day, such as legumes, iron-fortified cereals and breads, whole-wheat and whole-grain products, tofu, some dark-green leafy vegetables, seeds, nuts, tempeh, prune juice, blackstrap molasses, and dried fruit.

If your vegetarian diet allows you to consume eggs, keep in mind that they too contain nonheme iron. You can increase your body's absorption of nonheme iron by including a vitamin C–rich food with these nonheme iron sources at every meal, such as orange juice and other citrus juices, citrus fruits, broccoli, tomatoes, and green or red peppers. If you are a semi-vegetarian, eat a little meat, poultry, or fish with nonheme iron sources to help your body better absorb the iron.

Vitamin B$_{12}$

Vitamin B$_{12}$ is mainly found in animal foods. Because plant foods are not a reliable source of vitamin B$_{12}$, it can be a concern for vegetarians, especially vegans. Vitamin B$_{12}$ is important for helping the body make red blood cells and use fats and amino acids. It is also part of the structure of every cell in the body. The body only needs small amounts of vitamin B$_{12}$. Because it is stored and recycled in the body, a deficiency in the short term is not likely. Over time, however, a deficiency of vitamin B$_{12}$ can result in anemia.

Every day, vegans need to consume at least one (preferably more) servings of foods fortified with vitamin B$_{12}$, such as fortified breakfast cereals, soy milk products, rice milk beverages, or meat substitute products such as vegetarian burgers.

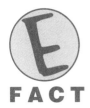

FACT

Some products, such as seaweed, algae, spirulina, tempeh, and miso, are not good sources of vitamin B$_{12}$ even though their packages may make a different claim. The vitamin B$_{12}$ that is contained in these products is inactive and is not in a form that the body can utilize.

If you are a vegetarian who eats dairy and eggs, vitamin B$_{12}$ intake should not be a problem as long as you consume the recommended number of daily food group servings. Vitamin B$_{12}$ is usually a standard vitamin included in most prenatal supplements. Most prenatal vitamin supplements contain cyancobalamin, the form of vitamin B$_{12}$ most easily absorbed by the body.

Zinc

It is tough to get enough zinc when you do not consume meat, poultry, or seafood of any kind. Zinc can be found in eggs and milk, as well as other dairy products. You can also get zinc from plant foods, though it is not absorbed as well as the zinc from animal foods. Zinc-containing plant foods include whole-wheat bread, whole grains, bran, wheat germ, legumes and peas, tofu, seeds, and nuts. Most well-balanced vegetarian diets supply enough zinc, but you should make sure that you consume sufficient amounts. Even mild deficiencies can have an effect on mental performance for both adults and children. Though your prenatal vitamin contains zinc, you should also be sure to get zinc from foods in your diet.

The Power of Protein

When you become pregnant, your protein needs increase by 30 percent. Protein can be found in both animal and plant foods, which makes it easy for both meat-eating and vegetarian women to get all of the protein they need. If you are a vegan, as long as you eat a wide variety of plant foods including whole grains, cereals, legumes, and soy products at each meal, you too should have no problem consuming all of the protein you need for a healthy pregnancy.

Protein is considered a macronutrient because it provides the body with energy, or calories. Protein is part of every cell in the body. Your body requires a constant supply of protein to repair body cells as they wear out. During pregnancy, you need protein to make new cells. Your body's tissues are all unique because of the differing amino acid patterns in their proteins. Amino acids are the building blocks of proteins. Your body uses about twenty different amino acids to make body proteins. Of those, nine are considered essential—your body cannot make them, and you must get them from the foods you eat. The others are considered nonessential amino acids because your body does make them as long as you consume enough essential amino acids and enough calories each day. Animal foods such as meat, poultry, fish, eggs, milk, cheese, and yogurt contain all nine essential amino acids. These foods are said to contain "complete proteins" or "high-quality proteins." Plant foods, on the other hand, contain essential amino acids, but not all nine together. These sources are said to be "incomplete proteins."

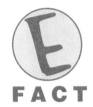

FACT

Soy is the exception to the incomplete protein rule. Soy is the only plant food that is a complete protein and contains all nine of the essential amino acids.

Gone are the days when vegans were instructed to eat foods in special combinations at each meal to make sure they were getting the right mix of essential amino acids to make proteins. Instead, vegans need only make sure they are eating a balanced diet that includes a wide variety of plant foods and that provides enough calories each and every day. If you are a vegan, this eating plan will ensure you are receiving all of the essential amino acids in needed amounts each day to make the proteins that you body needs. It is more important to think about your total day's intake rather than each meal individually.

Omega-3 Essential Fatty Acids

Fats are made up of two types: saturated and unsaturated. Unsaturated fats include monounsaturated and polyunsaturated. Two polyunsaturated fatty acids, linoleic acid (omega-6) and alpha-linolenic acid (omega-3), are considered essential because the body cannot make them. Omega-3 fatty acids are essential fats that can be very heart-healthy as well as vital to the development of a baby's brain and nerves. They are also vital to eye development, growth, and vision. In addition, researchers are studying the question of whether omega-3 fatty acids are helpful in preventing preterm labor and possibly protecting against postpartum depression.

Sources of Omega-3 Fatty Acids

Vegetarians are advised to consume omega-3 fatty acids from eggs as well as from plant-based ingredients such as canola oil, soybean oil, walnuts, walnut oil, ground flaxseed (which you can add to baked goods or smoothies), flaxseed oil, soybeans, wheat germ, and other nuts and seeds. For vegetarians who consume fish, fatty fish such as salmon, mackerel, herring, trout, tuna, and sardines also supply omega-3 fatty acids. If you consider a fish-oil supplement as another means of getting Omega-3 fatty acids, beware that some (those that come from the liver of the fish) can contain high levels of vitamin A, which in excessive doses may cause birth defects. Even though pregnant women need to be careful of how much fish and the type of fish they eat, keep in mind that not all fish contain toxic levels of mercury. Eating a few servings a week of allowed fish can help ensure your intake of Omega-3 fatty acids.

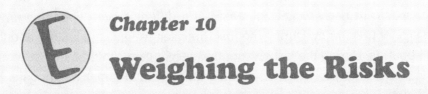

Chapter 10

Weighing the Risks

One popular question during pregnancy is, "How much weight did you gain?" Women tend to compare their weight gain with others', which can sometimes be frustrating and confusing. All women are different, and the rate and speed of weight gain will vary from person to person. Concentrate on what is healthiest for you and your baby by working closely with your doctor and following important guidelines.

Pregnancy Weight Gain

The health and weight of your baby at birth depend greatly on how much weight you gain over the course of your pregnancy. The weight of your baby factors into your weight gain, but your body also gains weight through its increase in blood volume—about 50 percent—as well as muscle, fluid, and tissue. Your body weight increases at a different rate depending on your stage of pregnancy. During the first trimester, weight gain is slow, about 2 to 4 pounds. During the last six months, weight gain should increase to about ½ to 1 pound per week, depending on your total target weight gain. Even though all women differ slightly, it is best to gain weight at a steady pace.

Trimester	Weight Gain
First trimester (1–3 months)	2 to 4 pounds
Second trimester (4–6 months)	12 to 14 pounds
Third trimester (7–9 months)	8 to 10 pounds

Your body weight before pregnancy will help to determine a healthy weight gain for you during pregnancy. The American College of Obstetricians and Gynecologists recommends the following target weight gains for healthy women. Keep in mind that these are only guidelines and that every woman is unique.

Pre-Pregnancy Weight*	Suggested Weight Gain
Normal weight (BMI of 19.8 to 26)	25 to 35 pounds
Overweight (BMI 26 to 29)	15 to 25 pounds
Obese (BMI greater than 29)	At least 15 pounds
Underweight (BMI of less than 19.8)	28 to 40 pounds

*BMI, or body mass index, according to National Academy of Sciences classification. See Appendix B for instructions on calculating your body mass index.

Because all women are different, suggested weight gains are expressed in ranges. Shoot for your target weight gain, and if you are not sure where your pre-pregnancy weight falls, speak to your doctor or calculate your pre-pregnancy BMI in Appendix B.

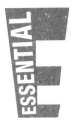

Women who are African-American or in their teenage years (younger than eighteen) are advised to gain toward the upper limit of the weight range to help decrease the risk for delivering a low birth-weight baby. Taller women should shoot for the higher end of the weight gain ranges, and shorter women (62 inches or under) should shoot for the lower end of the range for weight gain.

More Than One?

Multiple babies obviously means more weight gain. But remember, there is a vital need for the extra weight you need to gain! You are supporting more than one baby. Infants of multiple births have a much greater chance of being born premature or at a low birth weight. Women carrying twins are expected to gain about 35 to 45 pounds. Although women carrying triplets usually don't go full-term, if they did, they would need to gain somewhere around 50 to 60 pounds. Most women carrying twins have a higher-than-average weight gain in the first trimester. Experts stress the importance of early weight gain for women pregnant with twins because weight gain in the first two trimesters has been found to have the greatest impact on the birth weight of the babies.

Breaking Down Your Weight Gain

Your body is expanding. You know that not all of this extra weight can be coming from your baby alone, so where is it coming from? Many different parts of your body are used to support a healthy pregnancy, such as the storage of extra body fat to sustain the baby's rapid growth and provide needed energy during labor, delivery, and breastfeeding. It may ease your mind a bit to know exactly what is contributing to your weight gain and the importance of each component. The following chart will give you an approximate breakdown of a normal 25- to 35-pound weight gain. Of course, the picture differs somewhat from woman to woman.

Baby	7 to 8 pounds
Placenta	1 to 2 pounds
Amniotic fluid	2 pounds
Uterus	2 pounds
Breasts	1 to 2 pounds
Increase in blood volume	3 pounds
Body fat	5 or more pounds
Increase in muscle tissue and fluid	4 to 7 pounds

Weight Woes

Ideally, you will be at a healthy weight before you become pregnant and then gain the advised amount of weight during pregnancy. Unfortunately, this does not always happen. There can be consequences to gaining too much or too little weight over the course of your pregnancy. The baby's birth weight and/ or size at birth depends on your weight gain during pregnancy. Appropriate weight gain ensures a healthier outcome for both you and your baby.

Steady Now

Your goal should be to maintain a steady weight gain throughout your pregnancy. Your baby requires a daily supply of essential nutrients during your entire pregnancy, and that comes from what you eat every day. Expect your weight gain to fluctuate a bit from week to week and to gain more or less depending on the stage of your pregnancy. However, if your weight fluctuates too much or changes suddenly, that could be a warning sign. Be aware of some of the following red flags:

- Gaining more than 3 pounds in any one week during your second trimester
- Gaining more than 2 pounds in any one week during your third trimester

- Not gaining any weight for more than two weeks in a row at any time during the fourth through the eighth months
- Gaining more weight than you anticipated (given that you are diligent about sticking to a well-balanced, healthy meal plan daily)

If you experience any of these or other warning signs, you should contact your doctor.

Don't be obsessive about weighing yourself every day. Your weight can fluctuate too much from day to day to pinpoint possible problems this way. Instead, make regular doctor's visits, and weigh yourself at home every week or two to make sure you are on the right track.

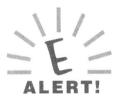

ALERT!

If you experience any sudden weight changes, including either a gain or loss, you should contact your doctor immediately. Sudden weight changes can indicate other problems that may exist.

Size at Birth Counts

An infant's weight and size at birth can be related to the risk of immediate health problems as well as to the risk of chronic diseases in childhood and adulthood. Although many factors can contribute to a baby's birth weight, the amount of weight a mother gains during pregnancy can definitely have a direct impact on an infant's size at birth. A baby who weighs too much or too little at birth can experience a number of problems.

Babies born weighing less than 2,500 grams, or about 5 pounds 8 ounces, are considered low birth-weight babies. Infants weighing less than 2,500 grams at birth may be premature (born before the thirty-seventh week of pregnancy) or full-term but "small for gestational age" (SGA) or "growth restricted." Babies can be premature but weigh more than 2,500 grams at birth. Some infants can be both premature and SGA. These infants are at even higher risk for problems linked to low birth weight. Technically, a baby is considered "larger than gestational age" (LGA) at more than 4,500 grams, or about 9.9 pounds, at birth.

Low birth-weight (or SGA) babies run the risk of developing more serious health problems as newborns, such as breathing and heart problems. They also have a higher risk for delayed developmental problems and learning disabilities later in life. Babies born at a low birth weight are more likely to experience asthma, respiratory tract infections, and ear infections. They are more likely to score lower on intelligence tests and to experience developmental delays. Those born weighing less than 2.2 pounds are at greater risk for cerebral palsy.

Infants born at an average weight and size run the least risk of problems as newborns and have the least risk of problems related to their size later in life. High birth-weight (or LGA) babies put both the mother and baby at risk for a more difficult labor and delivery. These babies can also have problems with low blood sugar and high blood counts at birth. LGA babies have a greater risk for carrying excess body fat during childhood and throughout adulthood.

Gaining Too Much Weight

It can be easy for some women to pack on the pounds during pregnancy. Even though you do need to gain some additional weight, gaining too much weight can have a negative impact. If you gain excess weight during pregnancy (usually more than 40 pounds), you increase your risk for gestational diabetes and high blood pressure. Both of these conditions can put you and your baby at risk for complications.

Too much weight can also make pregnancy much more uncomfortable, causing backache, leg pain, varicose veins, and fatigue. Gaining too much weight during pregnancy can also lead to a heavier baby, which can cause complications during labor and delivery. Some experts find that extremely overweight women tend to have longer labors and are at higher risk for cesarean sections. Additionally, according to the *Journal of the American College of Obstetricians and Gynecologists,* women who tend to gain more weight than what is recommended during pregnancy and who do not lose the excess weight within six months of giving birth are at a much higher risk of being obese eight to ten years down the road.

What to Do

It is wise to keep regular doctor's appointments so your health-care provider can monitor your weight on a regular basis. If you are gaining weight too rapidly, you may need to adjust your eating plan. Check to make sure you are not overeating or eating the wrong types of foods. Be clear on how many extra calories you should actually be eating, what portion sizes should look like, and the number of servings you should be consuming from each food group. Remember that you are not eating for two full-size adults. You only need to consume about 300 calories more than your maintenance calorie needs each day.

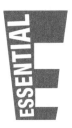

Do not take it upon yourself to diet or cut calories drastically to keep from gaining too much weight during pregnancy or to lose any weight you have gained. This can have detrimental health effects for both you and your baby. You need proper nutrition throughout your nine months for a healthy pregnancy.

Most importantly, do not obsess about weight gain. Keep in mind that you will gain and that you *need* to gain, but also remember this must happen in moderation. All women are different, so your rate of gain may differ from others. Stick to a healthy and well-balanced diet that includes all of the food groups in the correct servings and portion sizes; watch your fat intake; cut back on the junk foods; and get enough protein, fiber, and complex carbohydrates. Drink plenty of water, and exercise regularly. Do all this, and you are doing what you can to moderate your weight gain and stay healthy. If you are concerned about your diet, contact a dietitian who can help you properly analyze your food intake and put you on the healthiest path.

If you feel you are gaining too much weight, keep in mind that the gain may be due to water retention. Women who retain large amounts of water may experience swelling, or edema, in their lower legs and/or hands. In this case, you cannot really count on the scale to indicate whether you are eating enough or too much. Make sure you are drinking the recommended amount of fluids, which can help flush out stored fluid. Some degree of edema is normal, but if you feel you are experiencing an extreme case, speak with your doctor.

Gaining Too Little Weight

As gaining too much weight can be a problem, gaining too little can also cause problems. Not gaining enough weight during pregnancy can increase your risk for delivering a low birth-weight baby as well as preterm labor. Not gaining enough weight can come from improper nourishment. Not eating enough and not getting proper nourishment can deprive your baby of essential nutrients he needs for proper growth and development.

Some women may also experience little to no weight gain in the first trimester as a result of morning sickness. For those experiencing severe morning sickness, weight gain in the first trimester can be tough. Some women may even lose a little weight in the beginning of their pregnancy as their dietary habits change to healthier ones. Don't worry too much about not gaining weight in your first trimester. As long as you eat a healthy, well-balanced diet and consume the number of calories your body needs, your baby will be perfectly safe. What you don't gain in the first three months, you can easily make up for later on. It is important that you do begin to gain weight at a steady pace through your second and third trimesters. The ultimate goal is to gain the recommended amount of weight by the end of the pregnancy.

What to Do

If you are not gaining enough weight, the first thing you should do is talk to your doctor to make sure there are no underlying problems. If morning sickness is a continuing problem, speak with your doctor and a dietitian to learn helpful ways to get the calories you need. You need to assess your dietary intake. Make sure you are eating the correct number of servings from each food group, as recommended for pregnant women (described in Chapter 3). Don't skip meals or leave out food groups. Gaining weight doesn't mean you can eat anything you want. Eating junk food or fast food to gain weight is not healthy. You need to still make sure that all of your calories count. Some women who are underweight during pregnancy have a pattern of eating low-calorie foods and not enough protein. The following guidelines can help you to eat more healthy calories:

- Don't skip breakfast. Eat a healthy breakfast every day, and spread peanut butter on toast or add cheese to eggs to give you an extra boost of protein.
- Snack between meals on healthy foods to add calories to your day. Try snacks such as yogurt with fresh fruit, dried fruit, milkshakes, or cottage cheese.
- Add foods to your daily intake that are high in the "good" fats, such as nuts, seeds, fatty fish (in moderation), olive oil, peanut butter, and avocados. These foods can add lots of calories in just a small serving.
- Avoid junk food or fast foods that can add "bad" or unhealthy fats to your daily diet as well as too much sugar. Even though these foods add calories, most do not contribute much good nutrition.
- You may not need to eat more foods; instead, try to increase the portion sizes of the foods you already eat.
- Continue to be physically active. Exercise can help to stimulate appetite.

Dieting—A Dangerous Game

Pregnancy is not the time to worry about losing weight, no matter what your pre-pregnancy weight was. Nor is it the time to worry about spoiling your girlish figure. Once you become pregnant, your focus should be on gaining the recommended amount of weight and on living a healthier lifestyle for a healthy pregnancy. It is the time to eat healthy and stay fit, not skimp on calories. Your baby is constantly growing and needs constant nourishment. You can think about weight loss and reaching a healthier weight once your pregnancy is over and you have finished breastfeeding your baby.

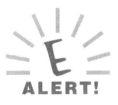
ALERT!

Never take any type of diet pill or weight-loss supplement, even those claiming to be "safe and natural," while trying to conceive or once you are pregnant. These can be harmful to the fetus.

Even when you are trying to conceive, it is advisable to stay away from extreme fad diets since you may not know you are pregnant immediately. Fad diets can be too low in the calories and essential nutrients you need from the very start of pregnancy. If you need to reach a healthier weight before pregnancy, do it by sticking to a low-fat, high-fiber, well-balanced diet and exercising regularly.

Dieting either before or during pregnancy can lead to nutritional deficiencies that can affect the proper development of your baby. Dieting by decreasing your caloric intake can lead to too-little weight gain during pregnancy, which can lead to problems such as premature labor and delivering a low birth-weight baby. Do not try to lose weight in order to keep from gaining too much during your pregnancy. Bigger women are unlikely to gain as much weight during pregnancy as smaller women might. Keep your weight gain to the advised levels, and do not try to lose weight!

Eating Disorders

Maintaining a positive body image can be tough for any woman. During pregnancy, body image concerns seem to become even more prevalent. Eating disorders such as anorexia and bulimia seem to be more prevalent in women and tend to peak around the childbearing years. For women who are already struggling with an eating disorder, pregnancy can be a difficult time that can cause the disorder to worsen. Any type of eating disorder can affect the reproductive process and be dangerous during pregnancy.

Types of Eating Disorders

Anorexia nervosa is an eating disorder in which a person starves herself by eating little to no food. These people have a strong fear of body fat and weight gain. The most dangerous hazard of anorexia is starvation and its extreme health consequences. Obviously, for someone who is pregnant and whose food intake is responsible for supporting a fetus, anorexia could be detrimental. Not eating during pregnancy deprives the baby of essential nutrients she needs for proper growth and development.

Bulimia nervosa is an eating disorder in which a person binges, or consumes a very large amount of food all at once, and then purges by forcing herself to vomit or by taking laxatives or diuretics (water pills). The dangers of bulimia nervosa include electrolyte imbalances from repeated vomiting. Many people with bulimia are able to maintain normal body weight, making the disorder more difficult to detect.

Binge-eating disorder is very common in women. With a binge-eating disorder, a person is unable to control the desire to overeat. These people are not necessarily overweight or obese. The food they binge on is usually not nutritious but instead filled with fat, sugar, and calories.

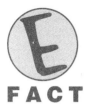

FACT

Eating disorders can affect fertility and reduce a woman's chance of becoming pregnant. Most women with anorexia do not have regular menstrual cycles, and about half of all women with bulimia do not have normal cycles. An irregular menstrual cycle can make it tough to get pregnant.

Effects on Pregnancy

Eating disorders can have a very negative impact on pregnancy. There are numerous complications that can occur and put you and your baby at higher risk. Some of these complications include the following:

- Premature labor
- Low birth-weight baby
- Stillbirth or fetal death
- Higher risk of C-section
- Low APGAR scores (the APGAR score is a quick evaluation of a newborn's physical condition after delivery)
- Delayed fetal growth respiratory problems
- Gestational diabetes
- Complications during labor
- Low amniotic fluid, miscarriage
- Preeclampsia (toxemia)
- Birth defects

Pregnancy can exacerbate other medical problems that are related to eating disorders, such as liver, kidney, and cardiac damage. Women who struggle with bulimia usually gain excess weight during pregnancy, putting them at higher risk for hypertension or high blood pressure. Women who struggle with eating disorders through pregnancy also tend to have higher rates of postpartum depression, and they can have difficulty with breastfeeding.

If a women abuses laxatives, diuretics, or other medications to help get rid of calories during pregnancy, she can cause harm to her baby in many ways. These types of over-the-counter medications can also rid the body of valuable fluids and nutrients before they can be used to nourish and feed the baby. Over-the-counter medications, even if they are considered safe during pregnancy, can be dangerous when used in this manner or when used excessively.

How to Cope

If you struggle with an eating disorder, you may be at an increased risk for several complications during your pregnancy. It is vital that you take action immediately to increase your chances of having a healthy pregnancy and a healthy baby. You can still take steps to help ensure a normal pregnancy. If you are able to eat healthily and gain the normal weight that you should throughout your pregnancy, you should have no greater risk of complications or birth defects than anyone else. Your first and most important step is to seek medical and psychological help with your disorder, if you have not already done so.

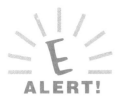

Even if you feel your eating disorder is a thing of the past, keep in mind that physical and emotional changes during pregnancy can trigger depression and a relapse of an eating disorder. Don't take it lightly. If you had an eating disorder in the past, talk to your doctor and consider visiting a therapist.

Follow some of these guidelines if you struggle with an eating disorder and want to become pregnant or have discovered that you are pregnant.

Before pregnancy, do the following:

- If you have an eating disorder and have not yet searched for professional help, that needs to be your first step—before you even begin to consider pregnancy.
- Achieve and maintain a normal and healthy weight.
- Consult with your doctor and receive a medical checkup. Ask about prenatal vitamins.
- Meet with a dietitian, and start a healthy pregnancy diet. Once you become pregnant, the baby will take from your own nutritional stores. If they are not built up, it could cause problems for both you and your baby.
- Continue any counseling, both individual and group, that you are involved with.
- If you have already gone through counseling, it would be a good idea to go back to your therapist to discuss concerns about body image that may surface during pregnancy.
- Seriously consider and discuss with your therapist the implications and complications of becoming pregnant before you have successfully recovered.

During pregnancy, do the following:

- Have a prenatal visit early in your pregnancy and discuss with your doctor your past and/or present struggles with eating disorders. The more honest you are with your doctor, the more he can help.
- Shoot to achieve an essential and healthy weight gain. The closer you are to a normal weight gain, the better chance of having a healthy baby.
- Continue to visit with a dietitian to receive instruction on eating a healthy diet, how many calories are necessary, and making the right choices. Seek out a dietitian with experience in eating disorders.
- Do whatever you can to normalize your eating and eliminate purging activities.
- Continue to seek counseling to address your eating disorder and any underlying concerns. A therapist can help you through the difficult times of your pregnancy when your body begins to change.

Just as important as before and during pregnancy is the care you continue to receive after your baby is born. Women with eating disorders are more susceptible to postpartum depression, so continue with your counseling. Eating disorder behaviors can also hinder your breastfeeding efforts, so don't allow yourself to fall back into unhealthy pre-pregnancy habits. To find out more information on eating disorders, visit the National Eating Disorders Association Web site, at *www.nationaleatingdisorders.org*, or the Renfrew Center at *www.renfrew.org*.

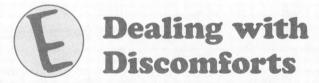

Chapter 11

Dealing with
Discomforts

Pregnancy can be a happy and exciting time, but unfortunately it also comes with some common discomforts. Some of these lousy side effects, such as morning sickness, backaches, and constipation, are extremely normal during pregnancy. Knowing how to deal with some of these discomforts can help make pregnancy more enjoyable.

Managing Morning Sickness

Even though that nagging feeling of nausea (and the vomiting that sometimes accompanies it) is commonly known as "morning sickness," it can occur at anytime of the day. Morning sickness is a very normal part of pregnancy, and its severity differs from woman to woman. It is thought to simply be a side effect of hormonal changes, particularly the pregnancy hormone HCG (human chorionic gonadotropin) and the change in estrogen. A woman's lifestyle can also affect the severity with which she experiences morning sickness. Women who do not get enough rest or are under more stress may experience more severe morning sickness. Though the experience differs greatly from woman to woman, for most, morning sickness begins in the fifth to sixth week from the first day of the last menstrual period (about the third week of pregnancy). For most women, morning sickness begins to subside at around fourteen to sixteen weeks.

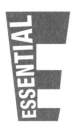

When morning sickness becomes severe, it is called hyperemesis gravidarum. It can cause weight loss, dehydration, ketone production (which is toxic to a fetus), and potassium deficiency. When a woman experiences severe morning sickness, testing may be done to rule out possible health conditions such as gastroenteritis, thyroid disease, cholecystitis (gall bladder), pancreatitis, hepatitis, ulcer, kidney disease, and fatty-liver disease as well as obstetric conditions such as multiple births and molar pregnancies. Notify your doctor if your morning sickness becomes severe.

Follow these suggestions to help decrease your symptoms of nausea and vomiting:

- Stay away from foods with strong odors or flavors that may trigger nausea. Women who are pregnant sometimes find that they have an exaggerated sense of smell, which makes common odors seem unappealing.
- Keep your kitchen well ventilated during cooking and meal times.

- Let someone else do the cooking for you.
- Go easy on spicy foods, such as those cooked with pepper, hot chili peppers, and garlic.
- Before getting out of bed in the morning, eat a starchy food such as dry crackers, graham crackers, melba toast, dry toast, pretzels, or dry cereal to help absorb and neutralize stomach acid. Carbohydrate-rich foods can help to slowly elevate your blood-sugar levels and help prevent symptoms of nausea.
- Get up out of bed slowly. Abruptly standing up from a prone position can increase feelings of dizziness and nausea.
- Instead of three large meals, eat five to six small meals or snacks per day every two to three hours. Don't allow yourself to become hungry. Nibble on carbohydrate-rich foods such as crackers, dry cereal, pretzels, and rice cakes.
- Drink beverages between meals, not with meals, and stay well hydrated.
- Limit fried, greasy, and other high-fat foods that may be hard to digest. Stick to easy-to-digest foods such as plain pasta, potatoes, rice, fruits, vegetables, lean meats, fish, poultry, and eggs.
- Eat your meals and snacks slowly.
- Before going to bed at night, eat a light snack such as peanut butter on bread and a glass of milk, yogurt, or cereal.
- Try beverages that may help settle a queasy stomach such as lemon or ginger tea, ginger ale, lemonade, peppermint tea, or water with a slice of lemon. Experiment with beverages. Some women do better with hot liquids, while others do better with cold.
- Choose foods that agree with you, and stay away from those that don't. Even if they aren't perfectly nutritious, it is better to get something in. If the problem persists, though, and you have a hard time eating nutritious foods for long periods of time, speak to your doctor and a dietitian.
- Take advantage of the times that you do feel good, and eat nutritious foods then, while you have the chance.
- Iron supplements and prenatal vitamins can sometimes intensify nausea. Make sure to take them with food. Do not stop taking them if you find they are adding to your nausea! Speak with your doctor first.

- Some women find relief by sucking on "fireballs," those intense cinnamon jawbreakers.
- Speak with your family and explain how important their support is for you during this time.

Gastrointestinal Complaints

Several gastrointestinal complaints can strike during your pregnancy. Knowing how to deal with them can help to decrease your discomfort. The way you eat and the lifestyle you live can go a long way in relieving some of these problems.

Controlling Constipation

Constipation can be a very common problem during pregnancy. Hormonal changes relax muscles to help accommodate your expanding uterus. In turn, this can slow the action in your intestines and the movement of food through your digestive tract. If you are taking iron from either an iron supplement or a prenatal vitamin, this can also cause constipation. Increased pressure on your intestinal tract as the baby grows can also cause hemorrhoids. Preventing constipation (as much as possible, anyway) can help you to avoid hemorrhoids. Some circumstances, such as hormonal changes and the growing baby, can't be helped, but there are plenty of dietary and lifestyle changes you can make that will make a difference.

Never discontinue your prescribed supplements. If you feel they are causing constipation or other problems, speak with your doctor before you stop taking them. Your doctor can recommend a different brand, maybe with a stool softener, or break up your iron dosages throughout the day.

A high-fiber diet can help to relieve constipation, but you must drink plenty of fluids or this option can make your constipation worse. Women under fifty should shoot for 25 grams of fiber daily. Make sure you are drinking eight to twelve cups of fluid daily. The majority of your beverages should be water, but you should also include fruit juice and milk in your total fluid intake. Include high-fiber foods to help alleviate your symptoms, such as whole-wheat breads and pastas, high-fiber breakfast cereals, bran, vegetables, fruits, and legumes. Some foods are known to act as natural laxatives, such as prunes, prune juice, and figs; other dried fruits may help as well. It is also essential to be physically active each day. Regular activity can help to stimulate normal bowel function. If nothing seems to help, speak to your doctor about possibly taking a fiber supplement such as bran, Metamucil, or a similar product mixed with water or juice once a day.

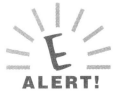

ALERT!

Do not use over-the-counter laxatives or stool softeners while you are pregnant to help relieve your constipation unless you have talked to your doctor first. Some may not be safe to use during pregnancy. Before relying on medications to relieve your symptoms, first make sure your diet, fluid intake, and activity level is adequate. Avoid castor oil as a remedy because it can interfere with your body's ability to absorb some nutrients.

Taming Gas

The same changes in a pregnant woman's body that cause constipation can also cause excess gassiness. Increase your fiber intake slowly and drink plenty of fluids each day. Increasing fiber too quickly, especially when you are used to a lower-fiber diet, can cause gas and other gastrointestinal problems. Some foods can exacerbate gas problems, such as broccoli, beans, cabbage, onions, cauliflower, and fried foods. Carbonated drinks can also cause problems with gas. All women are different as to what foods they can tolerate, so keep track of what bothers you so that you can cut back on those things.

Oh, the Heartburn

In the beginning stages of pregnancy, heartburn is usually due to hormonal changes. Heartburn has nothing to do with your heart but everything to do with your stomach and esophagus. The irritation you feel and the sour taste in your mouth comes from acidic stomach juices that back up into your esophagus. As your pregnancy progresses, your growing baby puts more and more pressure on your stomach and other digestive organs, which can cause heartburn. Although this problem can happen at any time during your pregnancy, it is more prevalent during the last three months when the baby is rapidly growing.

To help relieve symptoms, take the following steps:

- Eat small, frequent meals throughout the day, every hour or two if possible.
- Avoid known irritants that cause heartburn, such as caffeine, chocolate, highly seasoned foods, high-fat foods, citrus fruits or juices, tomato-based products, and carbonated beverages.
- Keep a food diary to track foods that might be triggering your heartburn. Everyone is different, so what bothers someone else may not bother you.
- Eat slowly and in a relaxed atmosphere.
- Do not lie down right after eating a meal. Instead, remain seated upright for an hour or two after eating. Even better is to walk after you eat to help your gastric juices flow in the right direction.
- Avoid large meals before bedtime.
- Limit fluids with meals, and drink them between meals instead.
- Sleep with your head elevated to help prevent acid backup.
- Wear comfortable, loose-fitting clothing.
- Talk to your doctor before taking any over-the-counter medications, such as antacids. Your doctor can advise you on what is safe to use.

My Pounding Head

Headaches can be very common in pregnancy, especially during the first trimester. The most common are tension headaches, which most people experience whether pregnant or not. If you suffered with chronic headaches before, they may become worse during pregnancy. Though experts are not sure why, the factor behind headaches in pregnancy is probably the crazy hormone levels and the changes in your blood circulation. The good news is that for most women, headaches during pregnancy will probably lessen—and maybe even disappear altogether—by the second trimester.

That is when the sudden rise in hormones stabilizes, and your body gets used to its altered chemistry. Other causes can include quitting your caffeine habit too abruptly as well as lack of sleep, fatigue, allergies, eyestrain, stress, depression, hunger, or dehydration.

Though most headaches during pregnancy are harmless, some can be a sign of a more serious problem. In the second or third trimester, a headache can be the sign of preeclampsia, a serious pregnancy-induced condition that includes high blood pressure, protein in the urine, and other indicators.

Relieving the Pain

The concern in pregnancy is over the products that can be used to relieve the pain of headaches. Most commonly used headache medications, such as aspirin and ibuprofen, are not recommended for use during pregnancy. Acetaminophen, or Tylenol, is safe to take but only as directed. Never take more than the bottle directs. In addition to over-the-counter medications, other remedies may help to relieve pain and should be tried first. For tension headaches, try a warm or cold compress applied to the forehead or back of the neck.

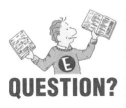

QUESTION?

When should I call my doctor about a headache?
If you are in your second or third trimester and experience a bad headache, or a headache for the first time during your pregnancy, you should contact your doctor. If you have a severe headache that comes on suddenly, won't go away, and is unlike any you have ever experienced, you should call your doctor. You should contact your doctor if you have a headache that worsens and is accompanied by vision problems, speech problems, drowsiness, and/or numbness. Also call your doctor if your headache is accompanied by a stiff neck and fever.

Pinpointing the trigger of your headache can help you to relieve it. If you are in a hot, stuffy room, get some fresh air. If the trigger is your screaming kids, drop them off with a relative or friend and take a break. Figure out what is triggering the problem, and try to defuse the situation. Take a warm shower or bath; if you have the time and money, get a professional to give you a massage and work out the knots. Since low blood sugar can be a trigger for headaches, make sure you keep your stomach full. Eat small meals every few hours so you don't become hungry. Avoid food that is high in sugar like candy, which can cause blood sugar to rapidly spike and crash. If possible, avoid fatigue and take daily naps if you need them. Regular sleep patterns can be very helpful in reducing the number of headaches you get.

Regular exercise can also help decrease the stress that sometimes causes tension headaches. Try to adopt regular relaxation techniques into your daily routine. Meditation and yoga can be very helpful in reducing stress and headaches. Find a professional to show you safe yoga and other relaxation techniques. Headaches can be caused by something you don't even realize is happening, such as eyestrain. If you find that after reading or sitting at your computer you get headaches, visit your eye doctor.

Even if you are a headache veteran, talk to your doctor about your headaches so that he can decide what type of treatment might be best for you during your pregnancy. Do not treat or diagnose yourself. If you have a headache that worries you, don't hesitate to call your doctor.

Migraines and Pregnancy

Migraine headaches are fairly common in women of childbearing age. About two-thirds of women who suffer from migraines before becoming pregnant note an improvement in their symptoms after the first trimester. This is especially true if their migraines were normally caused by hormonal changes during their menstrual cycle. Others, however, notice no change, and some even experience more frequent and intense headaches.

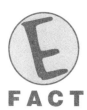

FACT

About 15 percent of migraine sufferers experience these terrible headaches for the first time during pregnancy, usually in the first trimester.

Migraines are much different than tension headaches. A migraine is a type of vascular headache that occurs when the blood vessels in the brain constrict and then dilate rapidly. Some people experience visual disturbances or an aura before the headache occurs. The pain is usually concentrated on one side of the head and takes the form of severe throbbing. Some people also experience nausea and vomiting as well as sensitivity to light and noise. Little is known about what causes migraines. The best way to treat your migraine headache during pregnancy is to try to avoid one.

If you are a regular migraine sufferer, you won't be able to take the medication that you were taking before pregnancy. You should talk to your doctor right away about what is safe to take so you know ahead of time what to do. When a migraine does hit, try to sleep it off in a quiet, dark room and apply a cold compress to your forehead or neck. A cold shower can help to constrict the dilated blood vessels. If you can't take a shower, at least splash some cool water on your face and the back of your neck.

Some migraines are triggered by certain foods. If you know what these foods are, avoid them. If you don't know, keep a food diary to try to pinpoint the culprits. Common offenders include foods containing MSG, red wine, cured meats, chocolate, aged cheese, and preserved meats such as hot dogs or bologna. As in treating other headaches, it is important to keep your stomach full and your blood sugar level up. Low blood sugar can also trigger migraines.

Try to stay physically active during your pregnancy. Evidence has shown that regular exercise can reduce the frequency and severity of migraines. Start slowly, though, because sudden bursts of activity, especially if you are not used to exercise, could trigger a migraine. Get plenty of rest, and adopt regular sleep patterns by going to bed at the same time every night and waking up at the same time very morning. Irregular sleeping patterns can be a big trigger for migraines. As with tension headaches, it is important to practice stress-relieving techniques.

Mouth and Gum Discomfort

Because of the hormonal changes that affect the blood supply to the mouth and gums, pregnancy can be demanding on your teeth and can make you more susceptible to mouth and gum discomfort. Increases in hormones can make your gums sensitive and make you more susceptible for gum disease such as gingivitis. Gingivitis is especially common during the second to eighth months of pregnancy and can cause red, puffy, or tender gums that tend to bleed when you brush your teeth. Having a sore mouth and gums can make it hard to eat certain foods, which can result in lower calorie intake or not eating from all of the food groups.

Taking Care of Your Teeth

It is important to see your dentist early in your pregnancy and to have regular checkups. Brush your teeth and tongue at least twice per day, and floss regularly. Chew sugarless gum after meals if you are not able to brush. Make sure you are taking your prenatal vitamins and calcium supplements daily, or as directed, to help strengthen your teeth and keep your mouth healthy. If you have any mouth or gum problems, see your dentist to keep them from interfering with your healthy diet.

If you experience problems with taste changes or recurring bad tastes, try using mouthwash. Often, chewing gum, mints, or hard candy can help lessen unpleasant tastes.

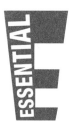

The taste of mint in toothpaste or mouthwash can trigger nausea in some pregnant women. If you experience this, try children's bubblegum-flavored toothpaste so that you can continue good dental care.

The Fluoride Connection

Fluoride is a trace mineral found in most tap water. It is known for its dental cavity-fighting properties. It also bonds with calcium and phosphorus to form strong bones. A baby needs fluoride in the second to third month, as her teeth begin to form. During pregnancy, the recommended intake is 3 mg, with a tolerable upper intake level of 10 mg. There is no need for a supplement as long as you drink or cook with fluoridated tap water. Bottled water usually does not contain fluoride. Fluoride is not widely found in food. Significant sources include tea, especially if brewed with fluoridated water, fish with edible bones, kale, spinach, apples, and nonfat milk.

Battling Leg Cramps

Muscle cramps, especially leg cramps, can be another bothersome discomfort during pregnancy. They usually surface late in the second trimester and in the third trimester of pregnancy. They can occur at any time of day, but they occur most often at night.

The truth is that no one really knows exactly why women experience leg cramps during pregnancy. Fatigue in muscles that are carrying around extra weight, as well as circulation problems later in pregnancy, can cause leg cramps. Some believe they are caused by excess phosphorus and too little calcium, potassium, and/or magnesium in the blood. Though there is no concrete evidence that supplementing with these minerals decreases leg cramps during pregnancy, some doctors may prescribe them anyway. The best idea is too make sure you are getting plenty of these nutrients by eating a healthy, well-balanced diet that includes all of the food groups. Some also believe that cramps can be due to inactivity, decreased circulation, and not enough fluids during pregnancy. Do not take any additional supplements unless you have talked with your doctor first. No matter what the reason, the good news is that there are ways that you can both prevent and alleviate your leg cramps. Here are a few tips:

- Avoid standing or sitting in the same position for long periods of time. That includes sitting with your legs crossed, which can decrease blood circulation in your legs.
- Stretch your calf muscles periodically during the day and especially before going to bed at night and when waking up in the morning.
- With your doctor's permission, take a walk or engage in some other physical activity every day to help the flow of blood in your legs and extremities.
- Stay well hydrated throughout the day by drinking eight to twelve glasses of water daily.

- Make sure you are getting plenty of calcium in your diet through food and prescribed supplements. Aim for three servings of dairy foods per day.
- If you get a cramp, massage the troubled area. You can also try applying a hot water bottle or heating pad to your leg. Straighten your leg and flex your ankle and toes slowly up toward your nose.

Do not go overboard with your calcium intake to relieve leg cramps. Consume no more than three dairy servings per day, and take your calcium supplement only as directed by your doctor. Too much calcium and phosphorus may decrease the absorption of magnesium, which also may be needed to prevent muscle cramps. Too much calcium over an extended period of time can also inhibit the absorption of iron and zinc as well as cause other problems. The upper tolerable limit for calcium is 2,500 mg per day.

Can't Sleep?

During the day, pregnant women seem to fight fatigue, but at night many end up fighting sleeplessness, especially during the first and third trimesters. During the first trimester, sleepless nights can be the result of endless trips to the bathroom due to increased need to urinate or from symptoms of morning sickness. Excitement, anxiety, and worrying about becoming a new mother can also disrupt normal sleep patterns. During the third trimester, physical discomfort due to the size of the abdomen, heartburn, backaches, leg cramps, and anxiety can all be culprits.

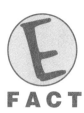

FACT

Don't be alarmed if you experience sleep disturbances during your pregnancy. With all of the emotional and physical changes to deal with it is no surprise that a reported 78 percent of pregnant women experience sleep disturbances such as insomnia.

If you experience insomnia, it may help to take afternoon naps—but not so many that you find it hard to sleep at night—to drink warm milk, or to take a warm bath before bedtime. Find ways to relax yourself to sleep, such as yoga, meditation, guided imagery, or reading before bedtime. Make sure your bedroom is at a comfortable temperature and that it is dark and quiet. Regular exercise during the day can also help. Above all, don't worry or get yourself all worked up about not being able to get to sleep. That will only exacerbate the problem. Do what you can to relax and fall asleep. Do not take sleeping pills or other herbal remedies without talking to your doctor first. If you feel you have a serious sleep disorder, talk to your doctor.

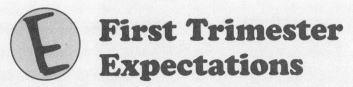

Chapter 12

First Trimester Expectations

Every stage of your pregnancy brings new experiences. As your baby grows and develops, you will experience different symptoms. Pregnancy affects every woman very differently. You can't even know for sure what symptoms will be a problem for you from one pregnancy to another. It will help to be prepared by knowing what changes your body will likely go through, how your baby is developing, and what nutritional concerns you should focus on.

Your Baby's Development

Pregnancy is generally divided into trimesters. Your first trimester of pregnancy ends at about twelve weeks, or three months after your last menstrual period. Your doctor may discuss your progress in weeks, which are measured from the first day of your last menstrual period—the day your doctor uses to calculate your due date and the baby's gestational age. Since it is usually impossible to pinpoint the exact date of ovulation and the date of conception, medical experts use your last menstrual period as the starting point for your next nine months. Basically, this means that the first week of your pregnancy is actually the week that you started your last period. Therefore, your baby can be up to two weeks younger than his gestational age. Every baby develops differently and at different rates in utero.

The First Month (1 to 4 Weeks)

About two weeks after the first day of your last menstrual period, your ovary released an egg into the fallopian tube. Your actual pregnancy began when that egg was fertilized by a sperm cell. In other words, you are not actually pregnant for the entire first month of pregnancy—weeks one through four.

Over the next week, the fertilized egg grows into a group of cells called a blastocyst. Once the blastocyst completes its journey down the fallopian tube, it implants in the uterus and divides into two parts. One half of the blastocyst attaches to the wall of the uterus and becomes the placenta while the other half develops into the embryo. This group of cells is already composed of different layers. The outer layer eventually becomes the nervous system, skin, and hair. The middle layer becomes bones, cartilage, muscles, circulatory system, kidneys, and sex organs. The inner layer becomes the respiratory and digestive organs.

The implantation of the egg into the uterus triggers the beginning of hormonal and physical changes. The amniotic sac, which cushions the fetus in the months ahead, begins to form. The early stages of the placenta and umbilical cord are visible and under rapid construction.

During the first month of pregnancy, the embryo looks like a tadpole. The neural tube, which will become the brain and spinal cord, starts to come together. A very primitive face begins to form, with large dark circles where the eyes will be. The mouth, lower jaw, and throat also begin to develop. The baby's blood cells are taking shape, and circulation will soon begin. By the end of the first month, the embryo is about a quarter of an inch long and is smaller than a grain of rice.

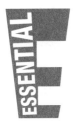

The placenta is the interface that provides all the nutrients the baby needs, including oxygen, and takes care of waste disposal. It also produces the hormones progesterone and estriol, which are produced to help maintain a healthy pregnancy. The placenta develops in the uterus just twelve days after conception.

The Second Month (5 to 8 Weeks)

You may not look pregnant yet, but by the second month of your pregnancy, plenty is going on. Major body organs are beginning to develop, including the heart, brain, kidneys, liver, intestines, appendix, lungs, and body systems. The baby's facial features continue to develop. The baby's ears, fingers, toes, and eyes begin to form. Tiny buds that will become the baby's arms and legs are forming. The digestive tract and sensory organs are now beginning to develop.

During this time, bone starts to replace cartilage. The baby's heart starts its contractions, which will become distinct heartbeats within the next week. The eyelids form and grow—though sealed shut—and nostrils begin to form.

The neural tube will eventually connect the brain and spinal cord, and by about the fifth week it closes. Blood circulation becomes evident at this time. The placenta and amniotic sac continue to develop. By the end of the second month, the embryo has started to look more like a person than a tadpole. It measures about 1 inch long and weighs less than $1/3$ ounce.

The Third Month (9 to 12 Weeks)

During your third month of pregnancy, the embryo has developed into a fetus. The baby is active, even though you may not yet be able to feel the activity. All major organs, muscles, and nerves are formed. The mouth has twenty buds that will eventually become teeth. The irises of the eyes are now forming. The liver, intestines, brain, and lungs are now beginning to function on their own. At around week eleven, it is possible to hear the "swooshing" sound of the baby's heartbeat for the first time with a special instrument called a Doppler sound-wave stethoscope.

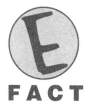

FACT

A Doppler stethoscope uses ultrasound to listen to the heartbeat of the fetus. The device is sometimes called a Doptone. The Doppler may be routinely used during your prenatal visits.

Several of the baby's ribs are now visible, and tissue that will eventually form bones is developing around the baby's head, arms, and legs. By the end of your first trimester, or third month, your baby is fully formed. Your little one has arms, hands, fingers, feet, and toes. Fingers and toes are separate, and they now have soft nails. Your baby's reproductive organs are developing, and the circulatory and urinary systems are working. The liver is producing bile.

Throughout the remainder of your pregnancy, the baby's body organs will mature and the fetus will gain weight, become longer, and fully develop. By the end of your third month, your baby is about four inches in length and weighs about 1 ounce. The most critical point of formation of the organs is finished, and your chance of miscarriage at this point drops considerably.

Changes in Mom

Along with changes in your baby's development, you will experience changes in your own body. The embryo secretes a hormone called chorionic gonadotropin (hCG), or the pregnancy hormone. This hormone triggers your first signs of pregnancy. In your first trimester, you may begin to experience nausea, vomiting, dizziness, headaches, a feeling of fullness or bloating, light cramping, constipation, poor appetite, frequent urination, and breast tenderness. You may need to go to the bathroom more often. This is because your growing uterus is pressing on your bladder and because hormones may be affecting your body's fluid balance.

Around week eight, your uterus grows from the size of your fist to about the size of a grapefruit, which can cause some mild cramping or pain in your lower abdomen or sides. Some of these problems will decrease as you continue on with your pregnancy.

Moodiness and anxiety can surface and make you feel like you are on an emotional roller coaster. Feeling happy one day and crabby the next is completely normal, due partly to fluctuating and very high levels of hormones. For many women, this moodiness and anxiety continues throughout pregnancy. You may begin to notice changes in your figure by the end of your first trimester. Your breasts have become larger, and you may notice that your waistline is beginning to expand just a bit.

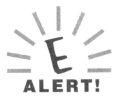

ALERT!

Weight gain in the first trimester should be about 2 to 4 pounds. Keep in mind that excessive weight gain during pregnancy can be a problem for both you and your baby. A normal weight gain during pregnancy, for women who begin at a normal weight, is 25 to 35 pounds. If your weight gain during the first trimester seems abnormal, speak with your doctor.

Worried About Lack of Appetite?

During the first trimester, a lack of appetite can be very normal. It is normal to experience nausea or morning sickness and to have a constant feeling of fullness that may cause you to eat less or just not want to eat. Don't make yourself too crazy about your lack of appetite—your good nutritional stores are nourishing the baby at this time. Even though you shouldn't worry too much, you should still do all you can to eat as nutritiously as possible. Follow the helpful tips given in Chapter 11 for dealing with morning sickness, such as eating small meals throughout the day, eating starchy foods before getting out of bed, and staying away from foods with strong odors.

Do the best you can to keep up your nutritional intake during this time, and keep in mind that by your second trimester these feelings should diminish.

Food Aversions

Food aversions during pregnancy are almost as common as food cravings. It is quite normal in pregnancy to suddenly be disgusted by the taste, sight, and/or smell of a certain food or beverage that you have always enjoyed. Food aversions can go as quickly and they come and differ from woman to woman as much as cravings do. Meat is probably the most common food aversion, though other popular aversions include water, coffee, tea, fried and fatty foods, highly spiced foods, alcohol, and eggs.

Why They Occur

Like food cravings, the cause of food aversions is pretty much unknown. There is some evidence that hormonal changes in pregnant women cause a heightened sense of smell, which may impact foods that are craved or avoided. Some speculate that food aversions are your body's way of telling you that you should avoid certain foods or beverages that are not good for you during pregnancy. Developing an aversion to coffee or alcohol can help you avoid something you shouldn't be having anyway.

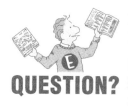

QUESTION?

Is it unhealthy to have an aversion to vegetables during my first trimester?

It is common for women to have food aversions even to healthy foods such as vegetables. Try drinking vegetable juice instead of eating whole vegetables. You can also eat more fruit, since many of them contain some of the same nutrients as vegetables. Keep taking your prenatal vitamins to ensure you are getting all of the nutrients that your body needs at this time. However, it's always best to get your nutrients from food before supplements. If you have a temporary aversion to a healthy food, make substitutions. If you're not sure what to substitute, be sure to speak to a dietitian.

On the other hand, some experts worry about aversions to foods that you should be eating and that can cause nutritional deficiencies. If you develop an aversion to specific healthy foods such as milk, make sure you try substituting something nutritionally similar such as yogurt. If you develop an aversion to water, it is essential that you do something to replace it. Try drinking water flavored with 100-percent fruit juice. Remember that food aversions come and go quickly. If you can't stand the sight of a food one day, make sure you try it again soon.

Fighting the Fatigue

Pregnancy, especially during the first trimester, can work your body overtime. It is normal to feel a little worn out when you are busy building another person! You may feel tired to the point of complete exhaustion. In addition to the obvious reasons for being tired, vomiting and/or lack of appetite can also zap your energy, as well as rob you of some essential nutrients. Hormonal changes in particular can cause fatigue. Being worried and anxious about being pregnant, along with frequent trips to the bathroom at night, can rob you of needed sleep. Most of these problems diminish in the second trimester, and you will feel much more alert. Feelings of fatigue usually surface again around the seventh month, when you are carrying more weight around.

You can't always completely fight fatigue, but you can give it a valiant try. Here are a few tips you can follow to help yourself deal with fatigue:

- Go to bed early and at a regular time to keep your body on a regular schedule. Shoot for at least nine to ten hours of sleep a night if your schedule allows it.
- Take short fifteen-minute catnaps during the day. Be careful of sleeping too much and interfering with your sleep at night. Your body will tell you when you need to rest.
- Keep as active as you can during the day with regular exercise. Even though you may feel too tired to even think about exercise, just a short walk during the day can help energize you.
- Take short breaks throughout the day to do some stretching and breathing exercises.

- Eat small, frequent meals throughout the day, and make sure you are eating a healthy diet that includes all the food groups. Eating throughout the day will fuel and help energize your body all day long.
- Stay hydrated by drinking plenty of water throughout the day, and make sure you have cut back on your caffeine intake.
- Eat energy-boosting foods, especially in the middle of the day. Include a good source of protein as well as carbohydrates, such as peanut butter on bread, grilled chicken and veggies on pita bread, chicken noodle soup, grilled cheese sandwich, or an egg white with cheese on a whole-wheat bagel.
- Good, energy-boosting snacks to nibble on during the day include dried fruit, fortified cereal and milk, yogurt with fruit and granola, cheese and crackers, nuts and/or seeds, frozen grapes or bananas, a granola bar, a milkshake, or vegetable juice.
- Don't be afraid to ask for help with household chores that may be zapping your energy, and do as many of your chores as you can while seated.
- Stay within your weight-gain guidelines. The more weight you have to carry around, the more fatigued you will feel.
- Ensure you are taking your prenatal vitamins, as directed by your doctor.
- If your exhaustion become debilitating or continues into your second trimester, speak with your doctor. Extreme exhaustion can be a sign of other problems such as anemia or thyroid problems.

Nutritional Concerns

The first trimester of pregnancy is most important for the development of your baby. Experts don't exactly understand how the mother and baby divvy up the nutrients, but we do know that the baby lives on the nutrients from the mother's diet and the nutrients already stored in her bones and tissues. The baby's health and proper growth are directly related to the mother's diet before and during pregnancy. It is essential for both you and your baby that you make sure you are eating a healthy diet and following the guidelines discussed in previous chapters. You should also be taking a prenatal vitamin at this time to ensure you are getting all of the nutrients that are essential to a healthy pregnancy, including folic acid, calcium, and iron. Good nutrition and a healthy lifestyle are essential throughout your entire pregnancy, though certain nutritional considerations may be more important at different stages along the way. In your first trimester, important nutritional considerations include folic acid intake, prevention of malnutrition, and dehydration.

Prevention of Malnutrition

Many critical nutrients play very important roles in the development of your baby, especially in the first trimester. As your baby develops, the demands on your body grow, requiring lots of extra nutrition. Because morning sickness often plagues women during their first trimester, malnutrition can be a nutritional concern during this time.

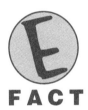

FACT

Malnutrition is defined as a state of impaired health caused by inadequate intake or inadequate digestion of nutrients. It can be caused by not eating a balanced diet, not eating enough, digestive problems, absorption problems, or other medical conditions.

Even if you are suffering with nausea and/or vomiting through your first trimester, you still should make every effort to find ways to eat as nutritiously as possible. The first trimester is a critical time for the development of your baby. Most women, even though experiencing these symptoms, will get the nutrition they need with a little effort and some helpful tips (described in Chapter 11). Women who suffer from excessive nausea and vomiting may deplete their nutritional stores and could become high risk for malnutrition.

If you have problems eating healthier foods or finding healthier substitutes during your first trimester, you should speak to a dietitian who can help you to ensure proper nourishment during this critical time. If you are able to eat but you still can't keep anything down, you should speak with your doctor immediately.

Dehydration

You need extra fluids in pregnancy for your increased blood volume and for amniotic fluid. Keeping properly hydrated can also help prevent urinary tract infections, constipation, and hemorrhoids, all common problems during pregnancy. Dehydration can be a concern in the first trimester if you are experiencing vomiting. Vomiting can remove vital fluids that your body needs to keep you in balance. Dehydration may also be a concern if you are not eating the proper amount of calories and if you are not drinking fluids due to feelings of nausea or fullness. If your doctor is concerned about dehydration, he may use a urine test to determine if you are maintaining a proper fluid level.

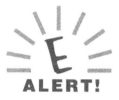

It is not unusual to be thirstier during pregnancy. However, being excessively thirsty can be a sign of other medical conditions, such as diabetes. If severe thirst is forcing you to drink large amounts of fluids, tell your doctor immediately.

You should aim to drink at least eight to ten glasses of fluids per day. If you are nauseated, fluids such as ginger ale or lemon tea can help soothe your stomach and contribute to your fluid intake. If you are vomiting, products such as Gatorade can help to replenish electrolytes. Some women who have a hard time getting plain water down do well with lemonade and/or juice. Stay away from caffeinated beverages—caffeine can act as a diuretic and compound the problem of dehydration. If you feel signs of dehydration, such as dry lips or a dry mouth, make sure you are drinking enough fluids. Be careful not to fill up on too many fluids at meals and not leave room for food. Drink your fluids between meals instead of with your meals.

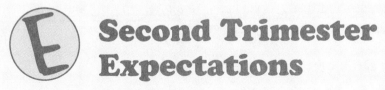

Chapter 13

Second Trimester Expectations

Congratulations, you made it through your first trimester of pregnancy! Your second trimester goes from week thirteen to week twenty-five (after your last menstrual period). There is still more to learn and experience. As your baby continues to grow, new experiences and symptoms will appear. As with your first trimester, it will help to be prepared for your second trimester by knowing what changes your body is going through and how your nutritional needs are affected during these months.

Your Baby's Development

By your second trimester, your baby is well developed. This stage of the pregnancy can be very exciting because you may start to feel your baby move at about eighteen to twenty-two weeks. If this is not your first pregnancy, you may even be able to feel movement earlier, at sixteen to eighteen weeks. Your baby looks like a small person now and is continuing to develop every week during this period.

Your Fourth Month (13 to 16 Weeks)

By your fourth month of pregnancy, your baby's fingers and toes are well defined. Eyelids, eyebrows, and nails are formed. Hair is starting to grow on top of the baby's head, and facial features are more prominent. The teeth and bones are becoming harder. The baby is moving her arms and legs and can even suck her thumb, yawn, and stretch. The baby is starting to now respond to outside stimuli. The nervous system is beginning to function, and the reproductive organs and genitalia are now fully developed. At this point your doctor may be able tell through an ultrasound if you are having a boy or a girl. The baby's heartbeat is now undeniably audible through an instrument called a Doppler. By the end of your fourth month, the baby is about six inches long and weighs somewhere around 4 ounces.

Your Fifth Month (17 to 20 Weeks)

During your fifth month of pregnancy, hair on the head, eyebrows, and eyelashes are filling in. A soft, fine hair, called lanugo, covers the baby's body. Meant to protect the baby, lunago is usually shed by the end of the baby's first week of life. Fat is beginning to form on the baby's body to help him stay warm and to aid in metabolism. The lungs, circulatory, and urinary systems are now in working condition. At this point, the retinas in the eyes are sensitive to light. The baby's skin is developing and appears transparent. Your baby can hear sounds such as your voice and heartbeat as well as sounds outside of your body. During this month, you may begin to feel the baby move as his muscles begin to develop. As the baby continues to develop, you will notice more movement. By the end of the fifth month, the baby is about ten inches long and weighs anywhere from 8 ounces to 1 pound.

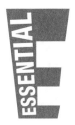

At this point, you should start sleeping on your left side because circulation is best that way. By the time you get to your fourth or fifth month, lying on your stomach or your back can put extra pressure on your growing uterus and may decrease circulation to the baby.

Your Sixth Month (21 to 25 Weeks)

During your sixth month, the baby is continuing to gain fat to keep its body warm. His or her growth rate is slowing down, but bodily systems such as digestion are continuing to mature. Buds for the permanent teeth are beginning to form, and the baby's muscles are getting stronger. The baby is very active and will respond to sounds and movement. The baby's body is becoming better proportioned. It is beginning to produce white blood cells that will help the baby fight infection and disease. You may begin to tell when the baby has hiccups by the jerking motions you feel. The baby's skin is more opaque than transparent and is wrinkled as the baby grows into it. The heartbeat at this point can be heard more easily through a stethoscope depending on the baby's position. By the end of the sixth month, your baby measures approximately twelve inches in length and somewhere around 2 pounds.

Changes in Mom

Some women consider this the easiest trimester of their pregnancy. The morning sickness and fatigue has subsided, but you haven't started experiencing some of the uncomfortable symptoms of the third trimester. By this time, you're finally starting to look pregnant, and you may need to begin wearing maternity clothes. You'll begin to feel your baby move during your second trimester. At first it may only seem like a fluttering movement, but as the trimester progresses there will be no question that you are feeling the little one move around. Other changes include an increase in blood volume to support the baby. This can give you occasional nosebleeds and bleeding gums and can make the veins just below your skin become more apparent. Increasing the humidity in your home will help to prevent nosebleeds. Your uterus is shifting, which will cut down on your need to go to the bathroom so much.

As the baby gets bigger, you may experience some common aches and pains, pelvic achiness, dizziness, heartburn, constipation, hemorrhoids, leg cramps, swelling in your feet and ankles, stretch marks, and backaches. Chapter 11 offers tips on dealing with some of these mild discomforts. During this trimester, your risk for bladder infections increases because the muscles of the urinary tract relax.

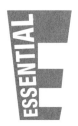

Urinary tract infections (UTIs) are among the most common types of bacterial infections during pregnancy. Bladder infections are at the top of list. Untreated, urinary tract infections can lead to dangerous kidney infections. Some women do not have symptoms at all. Others may feel a burning sensation while urinating, may have to urinate more often than normal, may have blood in their urine, and/or may feel like they have to go when they just urinated. To help prevent urinary tract infections, always drink plenty of water, urinate often, and don't wait a long time to urinate. If you feel you have symptoms of a urinary tract infection, see your doctor immediately.

Coping with Food Cravings

Though there is no agreed-upon explanation for them, food cravings are extremely common during pregnancy. There will be foods you can't seem to stomach, and there will be foods you just can't get enough of. Some experts blame raging hormones. Just as some women crave certain foods during their menstrual cycle due to hormones, the same thing happens during pregnancy. Some believe that in an opposite case from food aversions, the body's craving of a certain food signals a need for some nutrient or nutrients. Alternately, some scientists believe that cravings are the way the body takes care of getting its extra calories. Some of the most commonly craved foods for pregnant women include citrus fruits, chips, dairy products, spicy foods, ice cream, chocolate, and other sweet foods. In fact, women tend to crave sweet foods more during their second trimester than at any other time in their pregnancy. One thing is undeniable: A woman's taste preferences do change throughout her pregnancy.

Should You Give in?

Your food cravings may not necessarily be a problem or cause imbalances in your diet if you seem to be craving healthier foods, like fruit or milk. But what do you do when you are craving that hot fudge sundae? If high-calorie, high-sugar and/or high-fat foods are what you crave, you will have to exercise mind over matter on occasion. Giving in to cravings every time, especially if they are frequent and you are craving high-calorie foods, is a good way to pack on more pounds than you intended. In addition, if you seem to be craving and eating a lot of one certain food and not eating much of anything else, you may become deficient in important nutrients over time.

Do your best to fit your cravings into a nutritionally balanced diet. As long as you are eating a balanced diet and getting the essential nutrients you need for you and your baby, giving in to your cravings once in a while is probably fine. The bottom line is that indulging in your food cravings in moderation is harmless. You may find that your food cravings get less intense as your progress through your pregnancy.

Helpful Hints

Try some of these helpful hints to work cravings into your balanced diet:

- Eat a good, healthy breakfast. Skipping meals such as breakfast can increase the cravings for certain foods later in the day.
- Eat plenty of complex carbohydrates, such as whole-wheat breads, brown rice, whole-grain cereals, and pasta. Complex carbohydrates take longer to digest and therefore help to keep blood sugar levels consistent. Dips in blood sugar can cause cravings.
- Work the foods you crave into a nutritional diet. If you crave chocolate, try chocolate milk. If you crave ice cream, add sliced fruit such as bananas or strawberries your ice cream and give it a nutritional punch.
- Take a closer look at your total diet. Keep a food diary for a week or so and review it to make sure you are eating a balanced diet and getting the nutrients that you need.
- Indulge in your healthy cravings and try to find healthier alternatives to your unhealthy ones most of the time. For example, substitute nonfat frozen yogurt if you crave ice cream or pretzels if you crave chips.

- Think small when it comes to the portion sizes of your higher-calorie cravings. If you crave chocolate candy, instead of a whole candy bar, grab a one-bite serving.
- Stay active, and exercise regularly. Exercise can help curb hunger and tame cravings.
- Make sure you have the emotional support that you need. Pregnancy can put you on a mood-altering roller coaster, and these mood swings may cause you to turn to food for comfort.
- If you crave nonfood substances (see the pica discussion in Chapter 8) and cannot resist the craving, talk to your doctor.

Healthier Alternatives

There are always healthier alternatives that you can turn to when you crave certain foods. It is fine to indulge on occasion, but try healthier alternatives more often. Keep in mind, though, that even healthier alternatives in large amounts can add unwanted calories and pounds. Everything in moderation!

Instead of	Try this
Potato chips	Pretzels, popcorn (watch the butter), or baked tortilla chips
Ice cream	Nonfat frozen yogurt, sorbet, frozen juice bar, or sherbet
Colas	Instead of overindulging in diet sodas, instead try fruit juice or water flavored with a little fruit juice
Doughnuts	Whole-wheat bagel with low-fat cream cheese and/or jelly
Cake	Angel-food cake topped with fresh fruit
Apple pie	Applesauce with cinnamon
Cookies	Plain or cinnamon-coated graham crackers, vanilla wafers, gingersnaps, or animal cookies
Chocolate bar	Fat-free chocolate milk or hot chocolate
Cupcake	Reduced fat or fat-free muffin
Sour cream	Low-fat sour cream or plain nonfat yogurt
Cheesecake	Low-fat pudding or flavored low-fat yogurt
Sweets	Raisins or other dried fruit, fruited gelatin, flavored rice cakes

Losing Your Girlish Figure

In your second trimester of pregnancy, you will begin to gain more of your pregnancy weight. You should experience a steady weight gain of about 1 pound per week in your second trimester, although the rate of weight gain differs from woman to woman. Even though you may be losing your girlish figure, keep in mind that proper weight gain is a good thing in pregnancy. No matter how much some pregnant women hate to admit it, they struggle with their changing figures. Don't beat yourself up about feeling a little unhappy. It is very normal, and you should give yourself permission to experience both the joys and frustrations of watching your body change in so many ways.

Working on a Positive Body Image

Some women become upset every time they step on the scale and see the rising needle. If you worked hard to stay in good shape before pregnancy, pregnancy weight gain and the changes in their body can be tough to take. It is very normal for your physical self-image to fluctuate over the course of your pregnancy. The challenge for many women is to establish a healthy attitude and self-image about their changing weight and body image. During your first trimester, a positive self-image can be difficult when you always feel nauseous. However, by the second trimester, you should feel much stronger and healthier, making a positive self-image much easier to grasp. While many of the changes your body will go through seem to be beyond your control, certain strategies may help you to fully embrace the changes your body is going through and make your pregnancy a more positive experience.

Take Action

By working on a positive body and self-image before you even become pregnant, you can take much of the anxiety out of body changes during pregnancy. A positive body image is not about what you look like but how you feel about yourself. It is essential to remember this during pregnancy because you cannot control many of the changes in your body. Understand why your body is going through the changes that it is. Knowing that the changes are due to your growing and developing baby will make it easier to embrace them as positive. Maintain a healthy diet and caloric intake, and welcome the knowledge that you are feeding yourself and your baby with essential nutrients that will help her grow and develop properly. Failing to control your diet and giving in to the impulse to eat unhealthy foods can make you feel less in control and give you feelings of negative self-image. Instead of worrying about what extra calories will do to your body, begin instead to think of what they are doing for your baby's body.

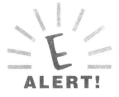

ALERT!

If you are not yet pregnant and you suffer from an eating disorder due to very negative body image, be concerned about recovery before considering pregnancy. Women with eating disorders can be at a much higher risk for miscarriage, pregnancy complications, and birth defects.

With your doctor's permission, develop a regular exercise program and stick to it. Women who exercise regularly during pregnancy maintain a higher self-esteem. Remaining active throughout your pregnancy can help lessen feelings of depression, stress, and worries over weight gain and body image. Define the attributes you find attractive in yourself and accentuate them to help make you feel better about yourself. Pamper yourself by doing things that make you feel good and that will help you to build your self-image. Keeping your weight gain within healthy, recommended limits can help make you feel better about your body size. Too much or too little weight gain can sabotage your efforts for a positive body and self-image. Most important, keep your eye on the prize at the end of the journey. Each time you begin to feel fat or your self-image seems to slip, think about that beautiful, healthy baby you are going to have. Keep in mind that this change is temporary. There will be plenty of time to regain your figure after your baby is born. Take a positive attitude and see the beauty and importance of the changes in your body. It is up to you!

Nutritional Concerns

As with your entire pregnancy, good nutrition and proper weight gain are essential during your second trimester. During this period, most women begin to experience decreased symptoms of morning sickness (though some may get morning sickness throughout pregnancy). It's a good thing these symptoms decrease for most because starting now, you need to begin to boost your calorie intake. The guidelines in Chapter 3 can help you to eat a healthy diet and properly add 300 calories each day. The nutritional concerns in this stage of pregnancy come from the digestive troubles that most women begin to experience.

As your pregnancy progresses into the second trimester, your baby continues to grow, which causes your stomach to work a little slower. Some women experience an intolerance to milk products at this time. Since calcium and other nutrients in dairy products are so essential to good health, especially during pregnancy, it is important to find an alternative. Guidelines in Chapter 8 can help you to deal with this problem. Other digestive problems women may experience as they enter the second trimester include gas, indigestion, and heartburn. Constipation can become a problem during the second trimester and continue until the end of your pregnancy. It is important to deal with these discomforts so that they don't interfere with your efforts to eat a healthy diet and don't turn into more complex complications. Tips and guidelines in Chapter 11 can help you to relieve these symptoms while still eating a healthy diet.

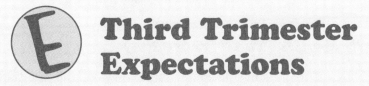

Chapter 14

Third Trimester Expectations

In the third trimester, you are starting down the home stretch! Your third trimester lasts from the twenty-sixth week after your last menstrual period until the birth of your baby, which usually takes place somewhere between the thirty-eighth to forty-second weeks. As with your first and second trimesters, it helps to be prepared for your last trimester by learning about the changes your body will likely go through, how your baby is developing, and what to expect at your doctor's visits at this stage.

Your Baby's Development

During your last trimester, your baby continues to grow larger, and his body organs continue to mature. Your baby is completing his development for his introduction to the world. With your baby growing and getting heavier, the last three months can get a bit uncomfortable—just keep thinking about the end result!

Your Seventh Month (26 to 30 Weeks)

Your baby will really start squirming around between the twenty-seventh and thirty-second weeks. Starting with your seventh month, the baby's lungs continue to develop, but they are not yet fully mature. To practice waking up Mom and Dad at all hours of the night, the baby begins to develop patterns of waking and sleeping. The baby's hands are active, and fingernails are growing. Muscle coordination is getting much better. The baby can now suck her thumb and can even cry. By week twenty-eight, the baby's eyelids are opening. The lungs are developed enough that if the baby were born prematurely, she would have a good chance at survival but would need to stay in a neonatal intensive care unit (NICU). Babies born earlier than seven months also have a chance for a higher survival rate with specialized neonatal care. As your seventh month progresses and the baby grows larger, he experiences a harder time moving around in the uterus due to space constraints. However, he still seems to find the room to do some kicking and stretching. The baby gains more fat on his body to help control his own temperature.

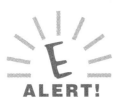

ALERT!

Around the seventh month of your pregnancy, it is normal for your blood pressure to increase slightly. However, you should contact your doctor if you experience severe headaches, blurred vision, or severe swelling in your hands, feet, and/or ankles. These specific symptoms could signal the beginning of a condition called preeclampsia, which is pregnancy-induced hypertension, or high blood pressure.

By the end of this month, the eyebrows and eyelashes are filled in and any hair the baby has on his head is becoming thicker. The head is now proportioned to the rest of the body. The baby's hearing is fully developed, and she can respond to stimuli such as pain, light, and sounds. Toward the end of this month amniotic fluid begins to diminish. Your baby now measures about seventeen inches from head to toe and weighs about 2 to 4 pounds.

Your Eighth Month (31 to 34 Weeks)

Starting with your eighth month, the baby is becoming too big to move easily inside the uterus. It may seem that the baby is moving less. The baby is developing more fat beneath his thin layer of skin, and he's starting to practice opening his eyes. Most of his internal systems and organs are now well developed except the lungs, which are not quite yet fully matured. The baby's brain continues to develop at a rapid pace. These weeks mark a ton of growth for the baby. During the last seven weeks, the baby gains more than half his birth weight. As the baby becomes larger, he begins to run out of room and takes the fetal position by curling up. By the end of the eighth month, the baby begins to move into a head-down position, although that may not be his final position at birth. Your baby now measures around 19.8 inches from head to toe and weighs about 5 pounds.

Your Ninth Month (35 to 40 Weeks)

By nine months, your baby's lungs are almost fully developed. She still doesn't have quite enough fat under the skin to keep herself warm outside of the womb, but she is working on it. By the ninth month, the baby begins to drop lower into your abdomen, usually with the head in a downward position. The brain has been rapidly developing, and the baby's reflexes are coordinated so she can blink her eyes, turn her head, grasp firmly with her hands, and respond to stimuli. Every day, the baby is taking on a rounder shape, developing pinker skin, and losing her wrinkled appearance. The baby is beginning to get antibodies from you that will help protect her from illness.

In this last month, the growth of your baby tends to slow down, yet he is still collecting fat under his skin and, therefore, putting on more weight. The toenails have grown to the tips of the toes, as have the fingernails, which have grown to the tips of the fingers. The baby's arm and leg muscles are stronger, and he is beginning to practice breathing and working out his lungs. By the end of the ninth month, your baby will drop farther into your pelvis, hopefully with head aimed downward to the birth canal, to prepare for delivery. The drop of the baby will help you breathe a little easier. Your baby's length at birth is about eighteen to twenty inches on average, and she weighs about 7.5 pounds. Length and weight vary greatly from baby to baby.

Changes in Mom

By your last trimester, you will have put on much of your pregnancy weight as your baby fully grows and develops. You should be gaining weight at a rate of about 1 pound per week. You will probably begin to feel some pain in the ribs as your baby grows and pushes upward on your rib cage. The pressure may also give you some indigestion and heartburn. You may begin to see stretch marks as your uterus expands. Your balance and mobility will also change as you get bigger. Throughout your last trimester, as your baby continues to grow, you will begin to experience some discomforts such as leg cramps, mild swelling of the feet and ankles, constipation, difficulty with sleep, shortness of breath, lower abdominal pain, backaches, and Braxton Hicks contractions. You may feel a more frequent urge to urinate again as you did in the first trimester.

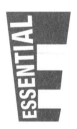

Around your twenty-eighth to thirtieth week of pregnancy, or even as early as twenty weeks, you may experience episodes in which your belly tightens, becomes firm, and then relaxes. This feeling, which is very normal, comes from contractions of the uterine muscles called Braxton Hicks contractions. They are a type of warm up or practice for the uterus for labor. Braxton Hicks contractions usually occur no more than four to six times per hour in your ninth month. If you can't tell the difference between Braxton Hicks contractions and true labor contractions, ask your doctor.

All women "carry" differently. Some will carry the baby higher or lower, bigger or smaller, wider or more compact. All these depend on the size and position of your little one, your body type, and how much body weight you have gained.

By your ninth month, your weight gain should be somewhere around 24 to 29 pounds. It may get more uncomfortable to sleep and move around, and it is normal to become moody and irritable. As you near the end, you may notice alternating feelings of fatigue and bursts of energy.

It is a good time to think ahead and prepare for your return from the hospital . . . with a newborn! Use those energy bursts to start stocking your freezer with foods you can easily pop in your oven or microwave. Cook casseroles, chili, soups, and other dishes that can be frozen and prepared later when you are too busy to worry about cooking.

Keep the Swelling Down

Moderate swelling or retaining of water in the hands, face, legs, ankles, and/or feet, known as "edema," is very normal in pregnancy. Edema is caused in pregnancy by the increase in blood volume and other fluids needed for the baby as well as from an increase in hormones. Ankles and feet tend to swell because the size of your baby and uterus can put pressure on the return circulation to your legs. The key is to get the fluids moving and to maximize the output of the kidneys. Edema can happen at any time during pregnancy, but it tends to begin around the fifth month and increase in the third trimester.

Moderate swelling is expected and normal in pregnancy as long as it is not accompanied by an increase in blood pressure and protein in the urine, which can be a sign of preeclampsia. Sudden or severe edema can also be a sign of this condition. If you experience these noticeable symptoms, contact your doctor immediately.

Here are a few tips for minimizing any swelling during pregnancy:

- Put your feet up, and elevate your legs whenever possible. Try not to cross your legs, which only makes circulation more difficult. Any time you can, get off your feet; the blood can circulate better and not pool in the extremities.

- Dress comfortably, and avoid wearing clothes that are too restrictive or too tight. That includes shoes that are comfortable and not tight or too high-heeled.
- Wear supportive hose or stockings that are specifically designed for pregnancy. Make sure you are fitted correctly.
- Avoid standing in one place for long periods of time. Move around to keep your blood circulating. Moderate exercise such as walking and stretching can be helpful.
- Minimize your time outdoors if it is hot and humid.
- Rest by lying on your left side as much as possible, and not just at night, but several times throughout the day for about thirty minutes.
- Drink water and fluids, at least eight 8-ounce glasses per day, to help keep your kidneys functioning properly and help flush out retained fluids.
- Don't consume excessive amounts of sodium. Avoid adding salt to foods and eating too many salty snacks or heavily cured foods.
- Visit your doctor regularly so she can monitor your blood pressure and severity of fluid retention.

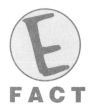

FACT

During the course of your pregnancy, your body will produce approximately 50 percent more blood and body fluids to meet the needs of your developing baby. The accumulation of these extra fluids accounts for almost 25 percent of a woman's weight gain during pregnancy.

Coping with an Achy Back and Legs

Backaches and leg aches can be very common later in pregnancy, as the baby begins to grow larger. By the second and third trimester, the weight of the baby on the pelvic bone can compress your sciatic nerve and result in pain along your back and legs. In addition to the weight of the baby and uterus, other causes of common aches include poor posture, hormonal changes (which can cause a loosening of the ligaments), and weak abdominal muscles. It is important to practice good posture with your pelvis tucked in and your shoulders back to relieve some of the pressure.

Ways to Relieve the Ache

Other tips that might help relieve the aches include the following:

- Wear low-heeled, but not flat shoes that have a good supportive arch.
- Do not lift heavy objects, such as children. If you have to lift something, bend at the knees, and keep your back straight. Use your legs to lift and not your back.
- Sit in chairs with good back support, or put a small pillow behind the lower part of your back.
- Try to sleep on your side with one or two pillows placed between your legs for support.
- Apply heat or cold to painful areas, or have someone massage them.
- Stay physically active to keep muscles toned and strong. Yoga stretches a few times a week may help relieve back pain, but make sure you learn how to correctly perform the stretches to avoid injury.
- Sleep on a firm mattress.
- Keep your weight under control with proper diet and exercise. Gain only the recommended amount of weight. Gaining too much weight will put even more stress on your legs and back.
- If back and/or leg pain is very bothersome, speak to your doctor. A licensed physical therapist may be able to help you ease your pain through postural awareness and safe exercises.

Dreadful Varicose Veins

Some women may get painful varicose veins during pregnancy, particularly if this problem runs in the family. The increase in blood volume, along with changes in hormone levels, and the increasing size of the baby and uterus can all add to the likelihood of varicose veins. The veins in your legs help to transport blood back to the heart and lungs for reoxygenation. It is a tough job, though, because gravity pulls the blood downward instead of up toward the heart and lungs. The leg muscles try to fight this gravity by contracting. As the muscles contract, blood moves through the veins where valves confine and hold it. If these valves become overwhelmed, which they often do during the later months of pregnancy, blood collects and stretches the vein walls out of shape. The painful result is visually swollen varicose veins. Support pantyhose can help to ease some of the pain. Put your feet up whenever possible, and avoid standing for long periods of time. Take a brisk walk every day to keep increase circulation. If your varicose veins become intensely bothersome and painful, talk with your doctor about other types of treatment.

Nutritional Concerns

Of course, good nutrition and proper weight gain are also essential during your third trimester. Too little or too much weight gain can become a more significant problem in this home stretch. Calcium intake is also crucial because the baby's bones are developing rapidly during the last trimester.

Weight: Walking a Thin Line

During these last three months, you can go either way when it comes to weight. The weight of your baby is increasing rapidly. For some women, this might mean that at meals, you feel fuller faster, making it difficult to get the essential calories that are still needed. If that's the case, it is best to try to eat smaller meals more often throughout the day. Snacks in between meals can help boost calorie intake. Choose a variety of snacks that will supply the nutrients that you need. If you have not gained enough weight throughout your entire pregnancy, you may not be able to make up for it all in the last trimester, but you can begin to ensure you are getting all of the calories that you need for a normal weight baby.

The flip side of the coin is gaining too much weight. You should be gaining about 1 pound per week during the third trimester. But by the ninth month, it is really the baby who is plumping up and not you. This is a good thing because the baby needs to be at a healthy weight by delivery. Low birth-weight babies have a harder time thriving and are much more susceptible to health and developmental problems. If by this time you are concerned that you have gained too much weight, discuss it with your doctor. If you feel you are gaining too much weight, do *not* restrict your caloric intake in hopes of losing a few pounds before the birth of your baby. In your ninth month, it is still important to eat a healthy diet and to pack a nutritional punch at each and every meal and snack. It is never too late to switch to a healthier diet for the proper nourishment of your baby and for a healthier weight gain. Eating a healthier diet can also help provide you with the important energy you will need for the delivery process.

Crucial Calcium

Although calcium is an essential nutrient before, during, and after pregnancy, it is especially crucial in the last three months of pregnancy. This is the time that your baby's bones and teeth are rapidly developing. If the baby can't get enough calcium from your dietary intake, he will take what he needs from your own stores. If your baby is relying on your stores of calcium for his needs, this can be detrimental to your health in the long run—for instance, by increasing your risk of osteoporosis. For this reason, it is vital that you get plenty of calcium through food and supplements in this critical third trimester. Chapters 1 and 4 can provide you with additional information on calcium.

Keep in mind that you can always overdo too much of a good thing, so watch that you don't abuse calcium supplements. You should not get more than 2,500 mg of calcium per day.

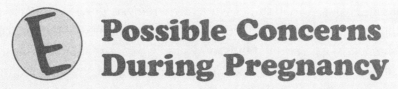

Chapter 15

Possible Concerns During Pregnancy

Though pregnancy is a happy and exciting time, health concerns can surface. It is important to understand what health problems can develop and to know the signs and symptoms to look for. You should always contact your doctor if you have signs and/or symptoms that seem abnormal to you or if you just are not feeling right. Listen to your body, and be aware of potential problems.

Hyperemesis Gravidarum

The majority of pregnant women experience some form of mild nausea and/or vomiting early in pregnancy. In fact, almost 50 percent of women experience some form of morning sickness. However, a very small percentage of women experience extremely severe and persistent nausea and/or vomiting. This is condition known as hyperemesis gravidarum (HG). This condition can make it difficult for a mother to consume the number of calories she needs, get enough fluids, and simply perform daily activities. If this condition is left untreated, it can lead to malnutrition, vitamin and mineral deficiencies, electrolyte imbalances, weight loss, dehydration, and even possible liver or kidney damage. These symptoms can all be damaging to the development of the fetus as well as to the health of the mother. When HG is treated properly, any adverse outcome to the baby—such as low birth weight, developmental problems, or prematurity—can be avoided.

Diagnosing

For some women, HG develops fairly rapidly within just a few weeks. For others, it may develop gradually over a period of a few months. Hyperemesis gravidarum is typically diagnosed through a thorough health exam, blood test, urine test, detailed health history, and the identification of symptoms characteristic to the condition including severe and persistent nausea and vomiting as well as dehydration and weight loss. HG is only considered as the final diagnosis when all other possible causes of severe and persistent nausea and vomiting have been ruled out. The condition typically begins in the period from week four to six and peaks between weeks nine and thirteen. Some women see significant improvements between weeks fourteen and twenty, while others may need significant care throughout the pregnancy.

Causes

The exact cause of hyperemesis gravidarum is not known. Though theories abound, none has yet been proven to be conclusive. Most likely, the condition is the result of more than just one factor. The factors may vary from woman to woman, depending on genetic makeup, body chemistry, and overall health. HG does seem to be more common in first-time pregnancies, women who are carrying more than one baby, younger women, obese women, and women who have had hyperemesis gravidarum in past pregnancies. Most theories focus on hormonal changes, such as an increase in estrogen and pregnancy hormone, physical changes, psychological causes, hyperthyroidism, gastric reflux problems, and nutrient deficiencies such as vitamin B_6 and zinc.

Signs and Symptoms

There are many different symptoms of HG besides the obvious severe and persistent nausea and vomiting. Additional symptoms may include rapid heartbeat, anemia, dehydration, vitamin and mineral deficiencies, weight loss of 5 percent or more from pre-pregnancy weight, ketosis, excessive salivation, extreme fatigue, headache, strong food aversions and/or cravings, heightened sense of smell, gallbladder problems, and low blood pressure. There can also be complications from extensive vomiting, such as gastric ulcers and esophageal bleeding, that can worsen ongoing nausea. For many women, this condition has a financial impact as well as an emotional and social one. It can begin to greatly affect the quality of life. Sufferers may not be able to work, complete daily household chores, or even care for young children. The earlier proper medical treatment is given, the better chance for a decrease in severity of symptoms and for a quicker recovery with no complications.

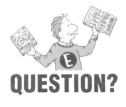

QUESTION?

When is morning sickness something more serious?
If you vomit more than three or four times a day, are hardly able to keep any food down, lose weight, feel very tired and dizzy, and urinate less than usual, you may have something more serious than run-of-the-mill morning sickness—specifically, you may be suffering from hyperemesis gravidarum (HG). Additional symptoms include increased heart rate, headaches, and pale, dry-looking skin. It is important to diagnose and treat HG as soon as possible, so contact your doctor if you feel any of these symptoms or feel that your morning sickness is more serious.

Treatment

If you are diagnosed with hyperemesis gravidarum, you may need hospitalization to restore fluids, replace electrolytes, and to administer medications if needed. Some treatment plans may also include vitamin and mineral supplementation. Depending on the doctor, you may not be given food by mouth until the vomiting stops and dehydration has been rectified. Instead, your food will be supplied through a feeding tube, and you will begin on food slowly. Proper nutritional intake is one of the biggest challenges and most important issues for women who suffer from HG. If you are not getting sufficient nutrients to meet your baby's requirements, your baby will take it from your stores. This can deplete your nutritional reserves very quickly, and it might take months or even years for you to correct these deficiencies. Vitamins, especially the B vitamins, can be depleted very quickly, and if they are not replaced can worsen the symptoms. With hospitalization, you can get the proper care that is needed.

Iron Deficiency Anemia

Anemia is defined as a deficiency of red blood cells or red blood cells having a decreased ability to carry oxygen or iron. There are different forms of anemia, such as iron, B_{12}, and folate deficiency. During pregnancy, the most common is iron deficiency anemia.

It is important to be tested for anemia during your first prenatal visit so that measures can be taken for treatment if you are found to be anemic. Even if you test negative for anemia at your first visit, the condition can develop as you progress through your pregnancy. This is especially true in the last three months when the baby is using a lot of your red blood cells for growth and development. Most doctors will test you at different stages throughout your pregnancy, including at your first visit, at twenty-eight weeks, once admitted to labor and delivery, and after delivery.

Diagnosing

A diagnostic blood test that indicates hemoglobin and hematocrit levels can help to diagnose anemia. If these levels indicate a problem, additional blood tests and other evaluation measures may be used to properly diagnose you. Possible complications that can occur if anemia is not treated include premature labor, slowing of fetal growth, complications of dangerous anemia from normal blood loss during delivery, and an increased susceptibility of infection to the mother after delivery. Just because you are iron deficient does not necessarily mean you are anemic. For anemia to actually be diagnosed, you need to have a severe depletion of iron stores in your blood, with low levels of hemoglobin as well.

Most women are provided with iron through prenatal supplements before and during pregnancy to help prevent iron deficiency. Eating iron-rich foods such as lean meats, fortified breakfast cereals, spinach, pumpkin seeds, beans, and dried fruits can also be very helpful.

Causes

Women at higher risk of anemia are those who are unable to eat a balanced diet due to morning sickness or hyperemesis gravidarum, who pregnant with multiple babies, and who have overall poor eating habits, including inadequate iron intake. Your iron needs increase by 50 percent in pregnancy due to an increase in blood volume. Especially if your iron stores were not optimal before becoming pregnant, your iron can easily get used up to meet the demands of pregnancy, and that can lead to the risk of anemia. Good nutrition and proper supplementation before becoming pregnant and during pregnancy is vital to help build up your stores of iron and prevent the risk of iron deficiency anemia.

Signs and Symptoms

Unless blood cell counts are very low, the signs and symptoms of anemia can be very subtle. Symptoms vary from person to person and depend on the severity of the condition. Some symptoms include fatigue and weakness, headache, dizziness, rapid heartbeat, pale skin, and labored breathing or breathlessness.

Symptoms of anemia can closely resemble those of other health conditions and/or medical problems. Never diagnose or treat yourself. Always consult your doctor for a proper diagnosis.

Treatment

Treatment for iron deficiency anemia is based on many factors, including the pregnancy, overall health, medical history, the type and severity of the anemia, tolerance for specific medications, procedures, and/or therapies, and the doctor's protocol. In general, most treatment for iron deficiency anemia includes some form of iron supplement. Some of these are time-release capsules, while others are taken several times throughout the day. The amount of iron provided daily is more than the usual recommended daily allowance. In general, most therapeutic levels prescribed for treatment are between 60 and 120 mg daily. Once the mother's hemoglobin levels return to normal for her stage of pregnancy, the normal recommended daily allowance is usually resumed.

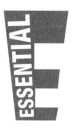

Iron absorption can be increased with vitamin C–rich foods and/or supplements. It is also helpful to take iron supplements between meals or at bedtime as well as on an empty stomach to help absorption. On the flip side, antacids can decrease the absorption of iron.

For many women, iron supplements can cause nausea and constipation. If these problems occur, ask your doctor about taking them with meals. Be sure you are drinking plenty of fluids, and increase your fiber to help relieve problems with constipation. If the supplements cause problems for you, do not stop taking them until you have spoken with your doctor.

Gestational Diabetes

Gestational diabetes mellitus (GDM) is a type of diabetes, or insulin resistance, that develops around the middle of pregnancy and ends after delivery. Women who are pregnant, have high blood sugar (glucose) levels and have never had diabetes before are said to have GDM. Gestational diabetes occurs when the body isn't able to properly use insulin or to make enough insulin to keep blood sugar levels in normal ranges, causing higher-than-normal levels.

Without enough insulin, or with the body not using it properly, glucose cannot leave the blood and be used for energy. GDM usually develops around the sixth month of pregnancy, or between the twenty-fourth and twenty-eighth weeks.

It can be unhealthy for both mother and baby if blood sugar levels are too high. Because GDM does not appear until later in the pregnancy when the baby has been formed, it does not cause birth defects seen in some babies whose mother had diabetes before pregnancy. If GDM is not treated properly or controlled, it can cause problems for the baby that include low blood sugar levels, jaundice, breathing problems, and high insulin levels. In addition, it can cause a baby to weigh more than normal at birth, which can make delivery more difficult and possibly necessitate a cesarean section. Babies born with excess insulin run a higher risk of obesity in childhood and adulthood, thereby putting them at higher risk for Type 2 diabetes later in life. GDM is different from other forms of diabetes in that it only occurs during pregnancy and goes away after delivery. Women who have diabetes before becoming pregnant are not classified as having gestational diabetes.

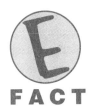

FACT

Gestational diabetes mellitus (GDM) affects between 3 and 5 percent of all pregnant women, about 135,000 each year. Women who have gestational diabetes during pregnancy are more susceptible to Type 2 diabetes later in life, though basic lifestyle changes may help lower this risk. Once a woman develops GDM in a pregnancy, the chances are 2 in 3 that she will develop GDM in future pregnancies.

Diagnosing

Some women do not experience any symptoms with gestational diabetes. Therefore, it is standard practice to screen most pregnant women at the twenty-eighth week of pregnancy. Women who are high risk for GDM are screened at their first doctor's visit as well as at twenty-eight weeks. The most common test used to screen for GDM is the 50-gram glucose challenge test. This nonfasting test measures the body's ability to use, or metabolize, glucose, the sugar that the body uses for energy. The test involves drinking a sweet, sugary beverage that contains a standard amount of glucose. A blood glucose test is taken one hour after the drink is consumed. Normal blood glucose values at the one-hour mark should be less than 140 mg/dl (milligrams per deciliter). If the blood glucose levels come out higher than normal, the results are considered abnormal and indicate the need for further testing.

Abnormal results after the one-hour screening do not necessarily mean a diagnosis of gestational diabetes. Instead, the next step is a three-hour oral glucose tolerance test (OGTT). This test involves fasting overnight (for about 12 hours) and is usually done first thing in the morning. The woman drinks a sweet, sugary beverage with a high concentration of glucose (100 grams). Her blood glucose levels are tested before drinking the beverage, which is a fasting blood glucose. After drinking the beverage, blood glucose is drawn every hour for three hours. If at least two of the blood glucose levels show up abnormal, a diagnosis of GDM is made. Early detection is important so that blood sugar levels can be controlled and complications for the mother and infant can help be prevented.

Causes

Gestational diabetes seems to stem from the placenta and its production of several hormones that help the baby develop during pregnancy. During the second and third trimesters, these "insulin-antagonist" hormone levels increase and can cause insulin resistance. Insulin resistance makes it difficult for the mother's body to properly utilize insulin, the hormone that manages glucose or blood sugar levels. This causes a higher-than-normal blood sugar level, or hyperglycemia. After delivery, these hormone levels, as well as glucose levels, return to normal.

Some women are at higher risk than others for developing gestational diabetes. Among this group are women with a strong family history of diabetes or a first-degree relative with diabetes, women who are obese, women who have had problem pregnancies in the past, women with a history of having babies more than 9 pounds at birth, women who have had gestational diabetes in past pregnancies, and women over the age of twenty-five. Also counted as high risk are women of certain ethnicities, including African-Americans, Latinos, Asian-Americans, Native Americans, and Pacific Islanders.

Signs and Symptoms

Gestational diabetes can be tricky because symptoms are not always obvious, and some of the symptoms may appear as normal symptoms of pregnancy. This makes screening for all women very important. Symptoms will vary from woman to woman, as each is an individual situation. Most of the symptoms that do appear are due to high blood sugar levels or hyperglycemia.

The most common signs and symptoms include the following:

- Increased thirst
- Increased urination
- Increased hunger
- Weight loss
- Fatigue

Less common signs and symptoms can also include:

- Blurred vision
- Frequent infections, including bladder, vagina, and skin
- Nausea
- Vomiting

Women who develop GDM during pregnancy are also at greater risk for problems such as high blood pressure and preeclampsia.

Treatment

If you are diagnosed with gestational diabetes, treatment needs to begin immediately. The goal of treatment is to help keep blood sugar levels within a safe range to help reduce the risk of complications to you and your baby during pregnancy and after delivery. Most women are able to keep their blood sugar levels within a safe range by eating a well-balanced diet that balances carbohydrates (55 to 60 percent of calories), protein, and fat. Regular exercise can also help to keep blood sugar levels in balance. Treatment should also include daily blood glucose testing. If a balanced diet and regular exercise are not enough to help control blood sugar levels, insulin injections may be needed. Oral glucose medications are not recommended during pregnancy.

Women with gestational diabetes should do the following:

- Eat smaller, more frequent meals throughout the day and not skip meals.
- Eat the required amount of calories and include all of the food groups each day.
- Eat a lower-carbohydrate breakfast because insulin resistance is the greatest when you first wake up.
- Eat a consistent amount of carbohydrates at each meal and snack.
- Add lean protein to each meal such as lean meat, egg whites, tuna, legumes, or nonfat dairy products.
- Choose foods higher in fiber, such as whole grains, legumes, fruit, and raw vegetables.
- Consume most carbohydrates from whole foods such as fruits, vegetables, legumes, and whole grains as opposed to sugary foods. Carbohydrates should not be overly restricted but should be moderate and spread throughout the day.
- Minimize intake of foods concentrated with sugar and saturated fats (animal fats). This doesn't mean you have to cut out all sugar, but you should moderate your intake.
- Drink at least 64 ounces of water daily.
- Be sure you are getting enough of all the essential vitamins and minerals each day.
- Exercise regularly in a way that does not cause fetal distress, uterine contraction, or maternal hypertension. Check with your health-care provider for instruction on safe exercise.
- Keep a steady and healthy weight gain.

There is no single way to treat all women with gestational diabetes. It is important that women work with their physician and a registered dietitian to help them develop an individualized treatment plan. If you develop GDM, it is important to keep in mind that you can still deliver a healthy baby. With the correct treatment and management of your blood sugar through life-style changes, you can have a perfectly normal pregnancy. It is important for you to be monitored on a regular basis by your doctor.

Hypertension and Preeclampsia

High blood pressure, or hypertension, occurs when there is a consistently higher-than-normal pressure or force of blood against the walls of your arteries. It is normal for a pregnant woman's blood pressure to drop during her first and second trimesters. By the third trimester, however, blood pressure usually returns to normal levels. However, in about 8 to 10 percent of pregnant women, instead of returning to normal, blood pressure begins to increase to abnormally high levels in the second or third trimester. This condition is known as pregnancy-induced hypertension. Women who enter pregnancy with high blood pressure are said to have chronic high blood pressure.

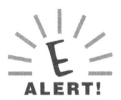

Mild hypertension during pregnancy is not necessarily dangerous by itself, but it can be a sign of a more serious condition called preeclampsia. High blood pressure puts a woman at higher risk for preeclampsia.

Preeclampsia, which is also sometimes called toxemia, is a disorder that only occurs during pregnancy and can also occur during the period right after delivery. It can greatly affect both the mother and unborn baby. Preeclampsia occurs in about 5 to 8 percent of all pregnancies, and very severe cases of preeclampsia can be life threatening. Typically, this condition develops after the twentieth week of pregnancy, in the late second trimester and into the third trimester, although for some it can develop earlier. High blood pressure that develops before the twentieth week is usually a sign of chronic high blood pressure or pregnancy-induced hypertension, but it can also be an early sign of preeclampsia.

Untreated, preeclampsia can cause high blood pressure, problems with blood supply to the placenta and fetus, problems to the liver, kidney, and brain function of the mother as well as the risk of stroke, seizures, and fluid on the lungs. Because the condition affects the blood flow to the placenta and fetus, the baby has a harder time getting the oxygen and nourishment it needs. These babies are often smaller in size and tend to be born prematurely. Women who develop severe preeclampsia can develop life-threatening seizures called eclampsia.

Both chronic high blood pressure and preeclampsia can develop gradually or suddenly and can be mild or severe. If you develop high blood pressure during your pregnancy, you will be monitored closely for signs of preeclampsia throughout your pregnancy.

Diagnosing

There is no single test that can diagnose preeclampsia. Your blood pressure is checked at each and every doctor's visit, which makes regular prenatal care even more essential for all pregnant women. A sudden rise in your blood pressure can be an early sign of preeclampsia. A urine test is also used to check for protein in the urine, which can be another warning sign.

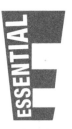

High blood pressure does not necessarily mean you have preeclampsia. In addition to high blood pressure, women with preeclampsia tend to have excessive swelling or edema in the hands and face as well as protein in the urine. Many women who experience high blood pressure during pregnancy without these other symptoms don't have preeclampsia.

Causes

The causes of high blood pressure and/or preeclampsia are not actually known. Preeclampsia seems to have a possible genetic link because women with a family history of the condition have a higher risk than those who do not. Preeclampsia is more common in first pregnancies as well. The risk of preeclampsia is much higher in women with any of the following conditions or characteristics:

- Carrying more than one baby
- Teenage mother
- History of preeclampsia
- Obesity
- Polycystic ovarian syndrome
- Over age forty

Other factors that put women at a higher risk include high blood pressure, diabetes, an autoimmune disease such as lupus, or a kidney disorder before pregnancy.

Signs and Symptoms

The signs and symptoms of pregnancy-induced hypertension and preeclampsia can be classified into three categories: mild, moderate, and severe. The signs and symptoms of high blood pressure and preeclampsia are often silent if the condition is mild. Suspicions usually surface unexpectedly during routine blood pressure checks and urine tests. Moderate preeclampsia can bring with it signs of high blood pressure, protein in the urine, rapid weight gain (more than 1 pound a day), problems with blood clotting, and excessive swelling of the hands and face. Severe preeclampsia can show signs of brain or certain body organ trouble, such as severe headaches, dizziness, vision problems, breathing problems, abdominal pain, and decreased urination. Very rarely, preeclampsia can progress to a condition called eclampsia that can be life-threatening, especially if the preeclampsia is not treated properly and early enough.

Signs of edema or swelling alone do not necessarily mean that you have preeclampsia. Edema can be a very normal symptom of pregnancy. It is considered more serious when it does not go away after putting your feet up, if it is very obvious in your face and hands, and if it causes a rapid weight gain of more than 5 pounds per week or more than 1 pound per day.

Treatment

If you are diagnosed with preeclampsia, treatment depends on the severity of your condition, the health of your baby, and the stage of your pregnancy. It is recommend that you lie on your left side as much as possible to help take unnecessary pressure off the blood vessels. This allows for greater blood flow.

If you develop mild preeclampsia close to your due date, and your cervix is showing signs of thinning and dilation, your doctor may want to induce labor. This will help prevent any complications that could develop if the preeclampsia were to worsen before your delivery.

If your cervix is not showing signs that it is ready for induction, your doctor will probably monitor you and your baby very closely until the time is right to induce or until labor begins on its own. If you develop preeclampsia before the thirty-seventh week of pregnancy, your doctor will most likely recommend bed rest, either at home or in the hospital, depending on your situation. For some, depending on the severity of the blood pressure, blood pressure medication will be prescribed until the pressure stabilizes or until delivery. With severe preeclampsia, a medication to prevent eclampsia (a very serious condition involving seizures) may also be prescribed.

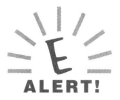

ALERT!

Even though cutting salt from your diet is usually a good way to help control high blood pressure, it is not a good idea to cut the salt in your diet if you have high blood pressure during pregnancy. It is essential that your body gets a normal intake of salt during pregnancy. If you have questions about salt intake with regard to your blood pressure, ask your doctor and a registered dietitian for advice and information.

In general, if you develop preeclampsia, delivery of your baby is the best way to protect you both from complications. If this isn't possible because it is too early in the pregnancy, steps will be taken to manage the preeclampsia until your baby can be safely delivered and survive outside of the womb.

At this point, early diagnosis through simple blood pressure checks and other routine tests at regular prenatal visits is the best way to detect pregnancy-induced hypertension or preeclampsia. The earlier the condition is detected, the earlier treatment and monitoring can begin and the better chance you and your baby have for a healthy pregnancy and healthy delivery.

HELLP Syndrome

About 4 to 12 percent of women who develop severe preeclampsia develop a condition called HELLP syndrome, usually in the last trimester. HELLP stands for the following:

- **H**emolysis (the breaking down of red blood cells)
- **E**levated **L**iver enzymes
- **L**ow **p**latelet count

Symptoms of HELLP include vomiting, nausea, headache, and pain in the right upper abdominal area due to problems with liver bloating. It is possible to experience this syndrome before the classic symptoms of pre-eclampsia even begin to manifest. Many symptoms of the HELLP syndrome are easily mistaken for the flu or for possible gallbladder problems. Some women develop HELLP syndrome without ever having preeclampsia, within two to seven days after delivery. Treatment for HELLP includes medication to help control blood pressure and medications to help prevent seizures and, occasionally, platelet transfusions. Basically, the only real cure for HELLP is delivery of the baby. Most women who develop HELLP end up delivering their babies early to prevent any serious complications. It is important to listen to your body, and if you have any of these symptoms, contact your doctor immediately.

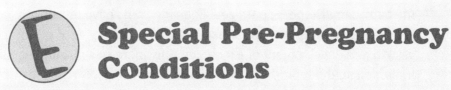

Chapter 16

Special Pre-Pregnancy Conditions

If you have preexisting conditions or are at a younger or older age and become pregnant, you may be worried about having a healthy pregnancy and a healthy baby. The success of your pregnancy will depend on your individual condition and your overall health before you become pregnant. The key is having your condition under control before becoming pregnant and being diligent in keeping up with doctors' visits, taking medications if needed, and following treatment plans during pregnancy.

The Teenage Mom

Even though they have steadily declined in the last ten years, teen birth rates in the United States remain high enough to be considered a public health problem. Pregnant teenagers are at a higher risk than healthy adult women for several reasons. Not only is the mother at risk, but the health of the baby can also be jeopardized. Teenaged girls have most likely not completed their own growth process. Adding pregnancy to a period of rapid growth and development of a teen certainly increases nutritional demands. In particular, the reproductive system is stressed as it is still in its own early development.

Risk Factors

Too often, teenage girls have poor eating habits and do not take daily multivitamin supplements. Coupled with higher nutritional needs, that can lead to possible complications. Other risk factors that can lead to a poor outcome for pregnant teens include the following:

- Extreme youth (younger than fifteen) and/or pregnancy less than two years after the onset of menstruation
- Poor nutrition or being under- or overweight before pregnancy
- Poor pregnancy weight gain
- Bad health, including infections, sexually transmitted diseases, preexisting anemia, smoking, or alcohol or drug use
- Poverty and lack of social support or appropriate healthcare
- Lack of general education and age-appropriate prenatal care and nutritional education in particular
- Rapid repeat pregnancies

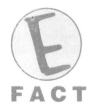

FACT

More than a million teenage girls become pregnant each year. About 485,000 of these pregnancies result in live births.

It is a known fact that pregnant teens are least likely, out of all age groups, to get the proper prenatal care. The earlier teens get prenatal care, the better chance they have for a healthy pregnancy, delivery, and baby. Pregnant teens are at a greater risk for complications during pregnancy including premature labor, anemia, and hypertensive disorders such as high blood pressure and preeclampsia. Unfortunately, teenaged mothers are also more likely to drop out of school and to experience financial hardship.

It is essential that teens get involved in childbirth education classes that are specifically developed for the teenage population. These classes can teach teens vital information concerning pregnancy, good nutrition, and a healthy lifestyle, as well as the processes of giving birth and the factors involved in being a parent. Classes like this can also act as a support group.

Special Nutritional Needs

Dietary intake is one of the most important and one of the most controllable factors for a healthier outcome for both the baby and the young mother. As with all pregnancies, adequate calories, protein, water, fiber, and all nutrients are essential for a healthy pregnancy. It is even more important that a teen ensures a healthy diet to support her growing baby as well as her own nutritional needs.

Pregnant teens who are at a young gynecologic age (the number of years between the onset of the menstrual cycle and the date of conception) or who are underweight and/or undernourished at the time of conception will have the greatest nutritional needs. Pregnancy is a period for rapid growth, and so are the teen years. During this time, a pregnant teen's body can compete with the fetus for nutrients. When nutritional deficiencies are corrected or—better yet—prevented, not only will the growth of the young mother and the fetus improve, but the risk of complications will decrease.

The additional calorie needs during the second and third trimesters of pregnancy for older teens is 300 calories per day. As a general nutritional guideline, teen mothers should consume between 2,500 and 2,700 calories per day during pregnancy. The notorious teen diet, made up of fast foods, soft drinks, and excessive sweets, can be very unbalanced. A nutritious diet should come mostly from a balance of all of the food groups each day.

Following the upper range of the number of servings from each food group in the Food Guide Pyramid can help teens to meet their needs.

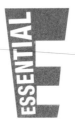

Teens have higher calcium needs because of their own growing and developing bones. In addition, their babies will demand calcium for developing bones and teeth. The teen mother needs 1,300 mg of calcium per day; she should consume at least three or more dairy servings per day.

As with adult women, each individual teen requires different amounts of foods that provide key nutrients to achieve the desired amount of weight gain and support of the pregnancy. Many of the same nutrients that are essential for adult women are also essential for teens during pregnancy, including folic acid, iron, calcium, and calories. An early prenatal visit is vital so the doctor can prescribe a prenatal vitamin as soon as possible.

The key concern with teens is that many have poor nutritional intakes to begin with and so do not have the nutritional reserves of an adult woman. As with adult women, the Institute of Medicine recommends folic acid intake of 600 mcg for teens during pregnancy. An adequate amount of folic acid very early in pregnancy is vital to helping reduce the risk of birth defects of the spine and spinal cord. Since many women, especially teens, do not know they are pregnant right away, it is best for all to consume at least 400 mcg of folic acid daily.

Iron needs increase from 15 mg before pregnancy to 27 mg during pregnancy for teens. Many females, especially teens, do not get enough iron through the foods they eat and many enter pregnancy with lower-than-optimal iron stores. Iron is essential, and needs increase during pregnancy due to the increase in blood volume of the mother. Iron is essential for making hemoglobin, the component of blood that carries oxygen through the body and to the baby. Low iron stores, in addition to a low iron intake, can lead to anemia. A prenatal vitamin supplement during pregnancy will ensure that a teen receives all the nutrients she needs in amounts optimal to boost the probability of a healthy pregnancy and baby.

Healthier Tips

Many of the same lifestyle tips that pertain to adult females also pertain to teens during pregnancy. The following are tips to eating healthier that can help to make a pregnant teen's diet a bit more nutritious:

- Don't skip meals.
- Prepare sandwiches and burgers with extra veggies, such as lettuce, tomato, or onion.
- Opt for grilled chicken breast instead of always choosing hamburgers.
- Eat whole-grain or whole-wheat breads, rolls, bagels, and crackers.
- Pile your pizza with loads of veggies such as mushrooms, green peppers, or sliced tomatoes instead of high-fat toppings such as pepperoni and sausage.
- Drink 100-percent fruit juice, fat-free milk, vegetable juice, or water more often than soft drinks or coffee.
- Eat fresh vegetables lightly steamed without butter or sauces.
- Bake, grill, or broil meats rather than frying them.
- Eat low-fat fruited yogurt or frozen yogurt instead of full-fat ice cream.
- Instead of French fries, eat baked potatoes with low-fat toppings such as salsa. When eating out, choose a vegetable or side salad over fries.
- Snack on fruit, vegetables, fruited yogurt, whole-grain bagel with peanut butter, pretzels, and other low-fat snacks instead of candy bars or cookies.

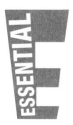

Even though many of the recommended nutrient intake amounts during pregnancy appear the same for younger women as for adult women, many of the recommended intakes for teens are lower than the adult's prior to pregnancy. This means that a teen's needs actually increase for many vitamins and minerals including calcium, vitamin C, vitamin B$_6$, biotin, and iron.

Weight Gain Is a Positive Thing

Many studies show that teens are less likely than older women to gain an optimal and safe amount of weight during pregnancy. Not gaining enough weight can increase the risk of many health problems for the baby, including low birth weight and developmental problems. Therefore, proper weight gain for pregnant teens is vital for a healthy pregnancy.

This can be a tricky subject for this age group because they are often worried about body image and deal with strong peer pressure. Eating disorders are especially prevalent among teenage girls. Some pregnant teens might be tempted to fight healthy pregnancy weight gain by drastically cutting calories or overexercising, both of which can do serious harm to the unborn baby. If a teen seems to have an unhealthy preoccupation with her weight, her doctor should be contacted immediately so proper and immediate intervention can be provided.

A teen at a healthy weight before becoming pregnant should gain between 30 to 35 pounds during the course of her pregnancy. For girls who are underweight before becoming pregnant, weight gain should be increased to 35 to 40 pounds. For teens who are overweight before becoming pregnant, weight gain should be about 20 to 25 pounds. Again, all teens are different, and each should discuss with her doctor the right amount of weight gain for her.

The Older Mom

As women become older, certain medical and obstetric problems can occur with pregnancy. Most women over the age of thirty-five have healthy pregnancies and healthy babies. However, they do face some special risks. In recent years, the birth rates for women in their late thirties to early forties has drastically increased. According to the National Center for Health Statistics, the birth rates for women aged thirty-five to thirty-nine and forty to forty-four years more than doubled between 1978 and 2000.

With recent advances in medical care, women who have babies later in life have a better chance for a healthier and safer pregnancy than in the past. All women should consult with their doctors before becoming pregnant, but this is especially important for older women who are planning to conceive and even more important if there are any preexisting health problems, such as diabetes or high blood pressure. Some of these conditions are more prevalent in women in their late thirties and forties than in younger women and can be risky to both the mother and baby. Proper medical monitoring and treatment before conception and throughout pregnancy can lower the risks and complications associated with these conditions and result in a healthy pregnancy and outcome.

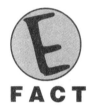

FACT

Fertility rates tend to drop slightly for women over age thirty-five. However, in general, many cases of infertility can be treated successfully.

Weighing the Risks

Studies do suggest that women over the age of thirty-five are at higher risk than younger women for complications such as high blood pressure, diabetes, and placental problems during pregnancy. They are also at a higher risk for miscarriages, stillbirth, and cesarean deliveries. As women become older, their chances also increase for having a baby with a birth defect or for chromosomal disorders such as Down syndrome, trisomy 18, and neural tube defects.

Fortunately, screening procedures are now available that indicate those babies who may be at an increased risk for these birth defects. Some of these screening tests include the Quad test, or maternal serum screen. Not all screening tests will screen for every birth defect. Keep in mind that these are only screenings. They do not provide a yes-or-no answer to the question of whether a baby definitely has a specific disorder. Instead, screenings will tell you the rate of your personal risk and whether you need further testing through a specialist. Remember also that just as a positive screen indicates a need for additional testing, a negative screen does not guarantee your baby will not be born with a birth defect. Additional diagnostic testing may include an ultrasound, amniocenteses, and/or chorionic villus sampling. There are pros and cons to these tests, and you should discuss them in detail with your doctor before making a decision.

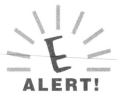

ALERT!

The American College of Obstetricians and Gynecologists recommends that women over thirty-five be offered specialized prenatal testing to diagnose or rule out chromosomal disorders such as Down syndrome.

Reducing Your Risks

You may not be able to decrease some of the risks that come with age and pregnancy, but by following the basic lifestyle rules for a healthy pregnancy, you can optimize the chance for a safer and healthier outcome. This includes visiting with a doctor before conceiving and addressing any preexisting medical problems as well as medications and immunizations. Taking a prenatal vitamin supplement prescribed by your doctor before conceiving is important to ensure you are getting all of the nutrients you need in proper amounts.

The Diabetic Mom

Many women begin pregnancy with preexisting problems, such as diabetes. In fact, about one in every 100 women of childbearing age has some form of diabetes. This includes Type 1 (insulin dependent) and Type 2 (noninsulin dependent) diabetes. In either case, most women with diabetes can have a successful pregnancy and healthy baby if the condition is well controlled. If you have diabetes, it is important for you to see your doctor before conceiving to discuss your care. You should have good control of your blood sugar levels for at least several weeks before becoming pregnant. This is because you might not even know you are pregnant until the baby has been growing for two to four weeks.

The baby's organs begin to form very early in pregnancy, and development can be affected by a mother's poorly controlled blood sugar levels.

High blood sugar levels early in the pregnancy can increase the risk for birth defects. Good control of blood sugar is just as important during the pregnancy as it is before pregnancy to decrease risk of other potential problems.

Weighing the Risks

If diabetes is not well controlled before and during pregnancy, problems that may arise include a higher risk of birth defects, a very large baby, pre-eclampsia, miscarriage, urinary tract infections, respiratory problems for the baby after birth, and too much amniotic fluid surrounding the baby, which can lead to preterm labor. Beyond possible problems for the baby, people who do not control their diabetes can end up with both short- and long-term health problems.

If you have diabetes, it is essential to meet with your doctor before you become pregnant. You may be advised to wait to become pregnant until you have your blood sugar under control. This can take time, so be patient. Your diabetes health-care provider needs to first determine if your diabetes is controlled well enough to decrease the risk for possible complications during pregnancy. A blood test, called a glycosylated hemoglobin test (HbA1c), is used to evaluate how well your diabetes has been controlled over the past six to twelve weeks. This blood test may also be used during pregnancy to monitor how well you are controlling your blood sugars.

Your diabetes health-care provider may also perform other tests before deciding that it is safe for you to conceive. These tests may include a urinalysis to screen for any possible diabetic kidney complications, a blood test to evaluate cholesterol and triglyceride levels, and an eye exam to screen for common diabetic problems including glaucoma, cataracts, and retinopathy. All of these tests can help your health-care provider determine whether your diabetes is under control. Your doctor will help you to properly monitor your blood sugar levels both before and during your pregnancy.

Reducing Your Risks

To better control your diabetes, you should monitor and record your blood sugar regularly, make necessary changes to your diet, take prescribed medications and/or insulin as directed, and exercise on a regular basis. It is also vital to achieve a healthy weight. Type 2 diabetes is very prevalent among people who are overweight or obese, and achieving a healthy weight often decreases or eliminates blood sugar problems. All these factors can lead to better control of your condition.

It is also important to take a prenatal vitamin that contains 1,000 mcg of folic acid at least one month or more before becoming pregnant. Women with preexisting diabetes are already at a higher risk for having a baby with neural tube defects, so folic acid intake is essential. A registered dietitian can work with you on your dietary intake as well as weight issues, which can both greatly affect not only your blood sugar levels but also the effectiveness of your medication or insulin.

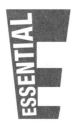

It is important for women with diabetes to continue closely monitoring their blood sugar levels following delivery because these levels might be more difficult to control. This can be especially true for women who breastfeed. Monitoring blood sugar levels frequently can help the doctor to adjust insulin doses back to pre-pregnancy levels.

Treatment Plan

If you have either type of diabetes, you should follow a diet and treatment plan during pregnancy that has been designed specifically for you. You should continue with nutritional counseling as your pregnancy progresses so that diet modifications can be made if necessary, and nutritional education can continue. Calorie needs during pregnancy vary among different women and depend on weight, height, stage of pregnancy, age, and level of activity.

However, most women require the standard 300 extra calories (after the first trimester), diabetic or not. If you are like most pregnant diabetics, following the Food Guide Pyramid and eating small meals throughout the day will help you gain the recommended number of pounds. Again, your meal plan will depend on your individual situation, including the insulin regimen that you are on. A dietitian can help you to plan out a diet that is right for you. Regular exercise, with your doctor's permission, can help to control blood sugar levels.

If you take oral glycemic medications to control your blood sugar, your [...] you to insulin for the time before you conceive [...] ral glycemic medications dur- [...] established and may increase [...] ts will generally change during [...] ulin requirements may decrease [...] the second half of pregnancy, [...] can create an increased need for [...] n may need insulin even if their [...] controlled with diet alone.

[...] sease include hypothyroidism and [...] ause thyroid disease often affects [...] omen to enter pregnancy with this [...] n have a completely normal preg- [...] ed properly and well controlled.

[...] been diagnosed with an underactive [...] roidism and had radioactive iodine or [...] ing thyroid hormone replacement. You [...] if you have had your thyroid removed [...] eplacement. The most common thyroid [...] include Synthroid, Levoxyl, Levothroid,

[...] conditions during pregnancy is close mon- [...] d be conducted every two to three months [...] The main thyroid function test performed [...] none). TSH is a chemical that is released [...] s hormone production in the thyroid. This by the p[...]

test can help diagnose and monitor hypothyroidism or hyperthyroidism. Also monitored would be T3 (Triiodothyronine) and T4 (Thyroxine) levels, which are both thyroid hormones within the thyroid gland that control the body's metabolism.

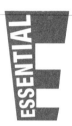

Thyroid hormone replacement medications should be taken at the same time every day. Antacids as well as iron supplements can make this medication less effective, which can be detrimental during pregnancy. Take prenatal supplements or any other iron-containing supplement at least two to three hours before or after thyroid medication. Most experts recommend taking thyroid hormone medication on an empty stomach and at least two hours after or one hour before eating to increase absorption.

It is important to get to the doctor for a thyroid function test as soon as you find out you are pregnant. You may need adjustments to your medication very early in your pregnancy. Until about week twelve, when the baby's thyroid gland is fully functional, you are the only source of thyroid hormones for both of you. A baby's thyroid gland will develop normally even if the mother's thyroid is underactive. If you are not getting a sufficient dosage of thyroid hormones early in your pregnancy, you can be at an increased risk of miscarriage, and the baby can be at an increased risk for developmental problems. It is perfectly safe for mothers to take thyroid hormone medication during pregnancy, and it is essential to take medications as prescribed throughout the entire pregnancy. There are no side effects for the mother or the baby as long as proper dosages are used. Women with a preexisting hypothyroid condition may need to have their medication dosages increased during pregnancy.

Dealing with Hyperthyroidism

Hyperthyroidism means you have an overactive thyroid gland, which can pose special concerns for pregnant women. The most common type of hyperthyroidism is called Graves' disease. It is important that hyperthyroidism be properly controlled during pregnancy because too much thyroid hormone can increase the risk for miscarriages, premature births, and birth defects. Uncontrolled hyperthyroid in pregnancy also increases the mother's risk for high blood pressure and heart problems. Because it can be tricky to treat hyperthyroidism during pregnancy, it is best for women with the condition to have it permanently taken care of before planning to become pregnant.

Antithyroid medication can be used during pregnancy but must be monitored very closely with examinations and blood tests because it can affect the baby's thyroid gland. These medications are used to cut down the thyroid gland's overproduction of thyroid hormones. The most common and safest type of medication used during pregnancy is propylthiouracil (PTU). Radioactive iodine, which is used to permanently treat the condition outside of pregnancy, is not safe for those who are pregnant because the baby's gland can be damaged. Antithyroid medication is the best form of treatment during pregnancy for hyperthyroid disease.

Asthma

Asthma is defined as a chronic respiratory disease that affects some 10 million American adults. Asthma is characterized by periods of inflammation or swelling of the airways, increased sensitivity of the airways to a variety of irritants, and obstruction of airflow. Many factors can cause symptoms of asthma to flare up, including allergies, irritants, infections (such as bronchial infections), exercise, weather, gastric reflux, and hormonal changes. This condition can be very manageable even during pregnancy and delivery with good medical care, monitoring, and medication. However, asthma can affect pregnant women in a number of different ways.

Some women experience an increase in symptoms, such as a greater number of attacks or an increase in the severity of the attacks. This is more common if the pre-existing asthma was severe or if asthma was worsened by a previous pregnancy. Most women notice no change in their symptoms, and a few may notice an improvement in their condition. Asthma that is not under control during pregnancy can threaten your health and your baby's. The goal of treatment should be to keep you and your baby healthy and breathing normally.

If you have asthma, you should have your condition under control before becoming pregnant. This means understanding how to deal with it and being aware of the causes for your asthma episodes. As with any pre-pregnancy medical condition, you should visit your doctor before trying to become pregnant. During this visit, make sure you have your condition under control, that all medications you are taking are safe during pregnancy, and that you know how your condition will be dealt with during the pregnancy. This is an opportunity for you and your doctor to develop an action plan. This will ensure a safer pregnancy and will cause less anxiety about your condition during pregnancy.

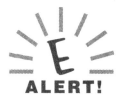

ALERT!

No matter what the severity of your condition is, treatment options and lifestyle changes should be discussed with both your attending doctor and your OB/GYN before you become pregnant.

Managing Asthma During Pregnancy

It is important to work with your doctor and your OB/GYN during your pregnancy to safely manage your asthma. Your breathing ensures an optimal oxygen supply for your baby. Working closely with your doctor will enable him to take the safest approach to treating your condition and to use the least amount of medication possible. Most of the drugs used to treat asthma are safe for use during pregnancy. As with any medication use during pregnancy, the benefits need to be weighed against the risks. Medications that may be used include preventers such as steroid inhalers, relievers or bronchodilators; long-acting relievers; and steroid tablets or injections. The type, frequency, and amount used will depend on your individual case and how frequent and severe your symptoms are. Uncontrolled asthma can be detrimental to a baby as well as the mother, and proper treatment often requires the use of medication. Sometimes it is simply a case of adjusting the dosage of the medication you are already taking to help control your asthma with minimal side effects to the pregnancy.

In addition to medication, other steps can be taken to control asthma, such as eliminating as much as possible typical allergens and irritants from your environment. Most people living with asthma are aware of their individual triggers. These may include pets, cigarette smoke, household dust, and environmental allergens such as pollen. Other triggers that may precipitate an attack include stress. It is essential to schedule and keep routine visits so that your doctor can accurately assess the respiratory function of both you and your baby. It is important to take your medication as directed.

Depression

Pregnancy should be a happy time in a woman's life, but many women struggle with depression while they are pregnant. In fact, about 20 percent of women suffer from depression during pregnancy, and 10 percent experience severe depression. Depression is a mood disorder that affects about one in four women at some point in their lives. Many times it is difficult to diagnose during pregnancy because it is assumed that symptoms are due to hormonal imbalances. Depression is an illness that can be properly managed and treated during pregnancy.

Mood disorders, such as depression, are biological illnesses that many times involve changes in the chemistry of the brain. During pregnancy, hormonal changes can affect the brain chemicals that are related to feelings of depression and anxiety.

Weighing the Risks

If untreated during pregnancy, depression can cause risks to the mother and the baby. It can lead to poor nutrition, weight loss, little sleep, drinking alcohol, smoking, illegal drug use, and/or suicidal behavior, which can lead to premature birth, low birth weight, birth defects, and developmental problems. Women who are depressed have a hard time caring for themselves properly, which can cause problems. Depression can arise during pregnancy, but it can also be a pre-existing condition. If you suffer from depression, it should be under control with therapy and medication, if necessary, before you consider having a baby. You should talk with both your doctor and therapist about your desire to have a baby. Depression during pregnancy can also put you at a higher risk for postpartum depression after the baby is born.

Signs of Depression

Signs of depression usually present themselves for two weeks or more. Some of these may include the following:

- Persistent sadness
- Difficulty concentrating
- Trouble sleeping or sleeping too much
- Loss of interest in activities that you usually enjoy
- Anxiety
- Feelings of guilt
- Negative self-image
- Reoccurring thoughts of hopelessness, death, or suicide
- Change in eating habits

Depression can be triggered during pregnancy by many different events, including relationship problems, history of family or personal depression, fertility treatments, previous miscarriage, stressful life events, complications in pregnancy, and history of abuse or trauma.

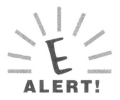

Never treat your depression with herbal supplements without speaking with your doctor first. Many herbal supplements, even though they are natural, can be harmful to your baby.

Treating Depression

First and foremost, if you feel you are struggling with depression, you should seek immediate help. Talk to your doctor about your symptoms and feelings. Your doctor can discuss the treatment options that will be the healthiest for you and your baby. Treatment options can include private psychotherapy, support groups, medication, and/or alternative therapies such as Reiki, light therapy, or touch therapy. If your condition is severe, your doctor may prescribe medication immediately. Medications proven to be safe during pregnancy include Paxil, Zoloft, and Prozac. As with any medications used during pregnancy, the benefits need to outweigh the risks.

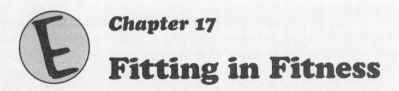

Chapter 17

Fitting in Fitness

Pregnancy is no excuse to sit back and put your feet up all day long! Research shows that regular exercise can greatly benefit women during pregnancy. It may not be the time to run a marathon, but a moderate version of your usual exercise routine can be safe and beneficial.

Benefits of Exercise During Pregnancy

Exercise has no harmful effects on a fetus and does not increase the risk of miscarriage or birth defects in a normal pregnancy. In fact, there is no doubt that if complications do not limit your ability to exercise during pregnancy, a regular fitness routine can be a big plus for both you and your baby. As with anyone and any exercise, you should be in good health before you begin an exercise program.

Many women exercise as an important part of their regular lifestyle. They want to continue throughout the pregnancy, which is possible with just a few moderate changes. Women who have never exercised before but want to begin adopting a healthier lifestyle can do so during pregnancy. These women just need to start out slowly with a mild exercise program. The level of exercise your doctor recommends for you depends on your level of pre-pregnancy fitness.

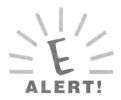

ALERT!

Regardless of whether you are a veteran or a first-timer, you should never begin an exercise program or participate in any regular physical activity without first discussing it with your doctor. Some medical conditions can rule out exercise for you. Your doctor will need to evaluate your overall health as well as any obstetric and medical risks you may have.

Benefits to Mom

Some of the benefits of a regular exercise program during pregnancy include the following:

- Reduces aches and pains
- Reduces constipation
- Reduces swelling and bloating
- Gives you more energy and stamina
- Builds muscle tone and strength
- Lifts your mood

- Improves posture, which helps with backaches
- Promotes better sleeping patterns
- Gives you a feeling of self-control, self-esteem, and confidence
- Gives you time to yourself
- Helps relieve stress
- Strengthens your cardiovascular system
- Keeps you from gaining too much weight (though it is not advised to exercise for weight loss purposes during pregnancy)

In addition to these benefits, regular exercise before and during pregnancy can help you to get back in shape faster after delivery. When done safely, exercise can have some wonderful benefits during pregnancy. If possible, a fitness routine should become a part of your healthier pregnancy lifestyle.

Exercise Not Your Thing?

Women who are not interested in regular exercise can obtain some of the health benefits of exercise simply by following a more active lifestyle. The key is to get your body moving every day. That can mean using stairs instead of elevators, washing your car instead of driving through the automated car wash, playing with your kids in the yard, or simply parking farther away from the store to get in a little more walking. Current recommendations from the Centers for Disease Control and Prevention (CDC) state that even short bouts of activity (ten minutes or so) several times a day can be effective in promoting some of the same benefits as regular exercise.

Playing It Safe

Exercise has many benefits, but use some common sense and know your limits to help keep you and your baby free from possible injuries. Changes in the body that occur during pregnancy can interfere with your ability to safely participate in some forms of physical activity. Even though there are many benefits to exercising during pregnancy, it is important to first make sure that it is safe for both you and your baby.

Pregnant women are able to participate in a wide range of recreational activities, though each activity and each individual should be evaluated for potential risks. The following are some general guidelines for pregnant women who have no additional risk factors, from the American College of Obstetricians and Gynecologists:

- You're encouraged to participate in thirty minutes or more of moderate exercise most days of the week, if not all days.
- During the second and third trimesters, avoid exercises that place you in a supine (on the back) position. Also avoid standing and being in a motionless position for too long.
- Activities with a high risk of falling or abdominal trauma may not be safe and should be avoided, including ice hockey, soccer, basketball, gymnastics, horseback riding, downhill skiing, and vigorous racquet sports.
- Scuba diving should be avoided throughout the entire pregnancy because it can put your baby at risk of decompression sickness.
- Exercise during pregnancy at altitudes up to 6,000 feet appears to be safe, but engaging in physical activities at higher altitudes can carry some risk.
- Pregnant women have less oxygen available for aerobic activities as they did before pregnancy, so don't expect to be able to do the same intensity as you did before pregnancy.
- Avoid activities or exercise that incorporate jumping or bouncing motions and sudden changes in direction because they can cause injury to joints and other areas.
- Don't overexert yourself to the point of breathlessness and/or exhaustion.
- Wear comfortable, cool, flexible, and supportive clothing as well as shoes. Wear a bra that fits properly and supports your breasts.
- Stay cool and properly hydrated by drinking plenty of water before, during, and after exercise.
- Do not become overheated, especially in your first trimester. Don't exercise on hot and humid days.

Some women may have medical and/or obstetric problems that would absolutely keep them from exercising. The American College of

Obstetricians and Gynecologists suggests that certain health problems are absolute contraindications to aerobic exercise during pregnancy, including the following:

- Heart disease or restrictive lung disease
- Incompetent cervix or ruptured membranes
- Pregnancy with more than one baby
- Persistent second- and/or third-trimester bleeding
- Pregnancy-induced hypertension or preeclampsia
- Placenta previa (in which the placenta grows low in the uterus and covers the opening of the cervix) after twenty-six weeks
- Premature labor during current pregnancy

If you have any of these problems or are pregnant with more than one baby, it is imperative to speak to your doctor before exercising. Other problems that may keep you from exercising, depending on your doctor's evaluation, may include severe anemia, chronic bronchitis, poorly controlled Type 1 diabetes, extreme obesity, extreme underweight, history of sedentary lifestyle, poorly controlled hypertension, poorly controlled seizure disorder, poorly controlled hyperthyroidism, and heavy smoking.

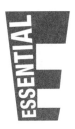

Most of the changes that the body goes through during pregnancy will last four to six weeks after delivery. Pre-pregnancy exercise routines may be resumed gradually after this point and as soon as your doctor deems them safe.

Developing an Effective Exercise Plan

The fundamentals of exercise remain basically the same for everyone, pregnant or not. You should develop an effective fitness plan that includes a warmup and a cooldown, with the activities of your choice in the middle. Once your doctor gives you the go-ahead to exercise, start exercising at a comfortable level that does not cause pain, shortness of breath, and/or excessive exhaustion. You should start slowly and increase your activity little by little, especially if you were not exercising regularly before becoming pregnant.

If you were an avid exerciser before pregnancy, you may need to make just a few simple adjustments in your program. You may find that you need to decrease your intensity level during pregnancy. The most effective plan is one that combines cardiovascular or aerobic exercise, strength, and flexibility exercises. It can be beneficial to find a variety of activities for your exercise plan because you might be more motivated to continue exercising throughout your pregnancy and beyond.

Warm Up and Cool Down

Warming up before you exercise and cooling down afterward is essential to an effective and safe program. Warming up for at least five to ten minutes revs up your body and gets your blood moving to prepare it for exercise. Cooling down for at least ten minutes gradually brings your heart rate and body temperature back to normal. You should never stop exercising abruptly without cooling down and slowing down your heart rate gradually.

Both a warmup and cool-down should include some light aerobic activity followed by gentle stretching. Stretching can help to maintain your flexibility, and prevent muscle tightening and injury during exercise. Stretching during your cool-down can also help to prevent sore muscles the next day. Stretching can be great any time of the day when you need to release some muscle tension.

As with other aspects of exercise during pregnancy, stretching may require some modification to avoid possible injury. During pregnancy, a hormone called relaxin causes your joints and ligaments to loosen, making delivery easier on the body. This makes it important to take some extra precautions when stretching. Stretching should always come after some type of warmup exercise that increases your circulation and internal body temperature. Stretching without first warming up can lead to pulled or torn muscles and/or ligaments. The key to stretching during pregnancy is to go nice and easy and never bounce. Do not push a stretch to the point of pain or past your natural range of motion. Hold on to a chair for support if you need to while performing certain stretches. Be sure to take full breaths while you are stretching to keep blood flowing through your muscles. Check out *The Everything® Pregnancy Fitness Book* for good suggestions of specific ways to exercise during your pregnancy.

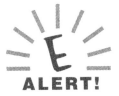

ALERT!

Standing motionless while doing prolonged stretches is not advised. This can decrease blood flow to the uterus as well as cause blood to pool in your legs, which can make you dizzy. Continue to move even when stretching by switching positions often or walking in place. Hold stretches for no more than fifteen to thirty seconds.

Aerobic Exercise

Aerobic exercise improves the fitness of your heart and lungs as well as your body's ability to use oxygen. When it comes to selecting a type of aerobic exercise that is best for you, keep in mind that all women are different. What works best for one woman may not work for someone else. Much of the decision will depend on your activity before becoming pregnant. You and your doctor should discuss what would work best for you. It is best to avoid exercises that incorporate excessive bouncing during pregnancy. Low-impact aerobics are a good alternative to high-impact exercise. Choose activities that are mild to moderate but take longer, as opposed to short-term strenuous exercise. The most comfortable and safe exercises during pregnancy are those that do not require your body to bear extra weight. Good examples include swimming, water aerobics, stationary biking, walking, dancing, yoga, and low-impact aerobics. Jogging and running can be safe, but they are better for women who were doing this before becoming pregnant.

Monitor your intensity by monitoring your heart rate while performing aerobic exercise. An easy way to monitor your heart rate is to make sure you can always carry on a conversation while you're exercising. If you can't, then you are exercising too intensely and should slow down. Modify your pre-pregnancy routine by decreasing both the length and intensity of your workout to avoid fatigue.

The best advice is to join a class for expectant moms that is lead by an expert in the prenatal exercise area. These classes can also act as a great support system for you and get you out to meet and socialize with new friends.

Strength Training

Weight training can definitely have some benefits as part of a regular exercise plan. It can help strengthen and tone muscles as well as build stamina. However, women who were not participating in a strength-training program before pregnancy are usually not advised to start during pregnancy. Strength training is definitely not advisable for all pregnant women and should be discussed with your doctor before you begin.

When using weights, it is important to use slow, controlled movements to help avoid injury to loosened joints and ligaments. Machines are generally preferred to free weights during pregnancy because they are more easily controlled. It is advisable to work with lighter weights than you might normally use and to compensate for the lower weight by doing more repetitions. It is important to breathe normally during strength training and avoid holding your breath so your baby continues to receive optimal amounts of oxygen. As with any exercise at this time, discontinue any strength exercise that causes pain or discomfort.

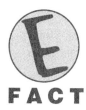

FACT

Avoid exercising the same muscles for two days in a row. Your muscles need time to recover. To see results, you only need to perform strength-training exercises for thirty minutes two to three days per week.

Starting with your second trimester, you should avoid lifting weights while standing. Blood can pool in your legs and cause you to feel lightheaded or dizzy. You should always avoid lying on a bench to lift weights or being in a position that leaves your abdominal area vulnerable to a falling weight. Most important, it is best to exercise safely, to use common sense if weight-training during pregnancy, and to discuss your program with your doctor before you begin.

Nutritional Needs

All of the same nutritional requirements that apply to pregnant women apply to the exercising moms-to-be. Pregnancy requires additional healthy calories, and these are even more important if you exercise regularly. You need to eat enough to support your pregnancy, your own needs, and the demands of your exercise program. The key is consuming enough calories to ensure an adequate weight gain.

Your exercise plan should include an eating plan that keeps you from exercising on a completely empty stomach or an overly full stomach. Eat something light at least an hour before you exercise to keep your blood sugar levels from dropping too low. A quick snack after exercise can also help to reenergize you and regulate your blood sugar levels. Make your pre-exercise snacks healthy ones by avoiding sugary or high-fat foods. Stick to foods such as high-fiber starches, lean proteins, and fat-free dairy products.

Walking for Health

Walking can be a great low-impact aerobic activity during pregnancy. It is an exercise that is safe, easy to do, and inexpensive. If the weather is less than optimal, you can try a treadmill or roam around your local shopping mall. You can vary the pace, add moderate hills, and add distance when you need too. As with any exercise, you should start slow and increase your pace and distance as you feel you can. You can add a warmup by walking slowly for the first five minutes and add a cool-down by using five minutes at the end to gradually decrease your pace.

Follow some of these tips for an effective walking program:

- Watch your posture as you walk. Stand up straight, lead with your chest, and use your abdominal muscles to support your back.
- Look ahead at the ground a few steps ahead of you and not straight down, which can strain your neck and spoil your posture.
- Get your arms moving to give your walk an extra cardiovascular kick. Move your arms from the shoulders, and don't swing them higher than your chest or across your body's midpoint.

- Take small strides. Long ones can hurt your hips and pelvic area, which are usually loosened by pregnancy hormones during pregnancy.
- Use a pace that is comfortable for your stage of pregnancy and keeps your heart rate at a safe and steady beat. Don't try to conquer steep hills that may send your heart rate soaring and put undue stress on your back.
- Invest in good athletic walking shoes that are comfortable, supportive, and fit your feet properly. If you have some swelling in your feet, you may need a larger size than usual.
- Avoid uneven terrain, such as beaches and trails, since your center of balance will shift as you become larger and you are more prone to fall. Avoid other dangerous terrain such as ice or wet pavement.
- If the weather outside is too hot and humid, opt to use an indoor treadmill, or walk at the mall.
- Find a walking partner. It can make walking more fun and can also be a safety net if something happens while you were walking.

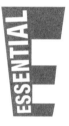

Your center of gravity shifts during pregnancy. This makes it necessary to take extra precautions when changing positions such as getting up from the floor, exercise equipment, or from a chair. Getting up too quickly can make you dizzy and cause you to lose your balance, so move slowly.

Know Your Limits

Part of a safe exercise program is knowing your limits. You need to pay attention to your body's signals and stop when your body is telling you to stop. It's not good for you or your baby to exercise to the point of exhaustion, breathlessness, or overheating. Warning signs that tell you to stop exercising and/or call your doctor include the following:

- Vaginal bleeding or amniotic fluid leakage
- Preterm labor or decreased fetal movement
- Dizziness or fainting, muscle weakness, or difficult or labored breathing prior to exertion

- Increased swelling in hands, feet, and/or ankles
- Headache, chest pain, calf pain or swelling
- Vomiting, nausea, or abdominal pain

Yeah for Yoga

Yoga can be a great exercise for flexibility, relaxation, muscle tone, posture, balance, breathing control, and developing concentration. All of these factors can help during pregnancy and again during delivery. Yoga combined with a low-impact cardiovascular exercise such as walking can round out a great exercise program. You can join a pregnancy yoga class or pick up a video specifically made for pregnant women. If you have never tried yoga before, be sure to start at the beginners' level. Yoga can be done at all different intensity levels, but while you are pregnant, you should concentrate on poses that are soothing, gentle, and fun. You want to make sure you avoid supine positions, or positions on your back, after the third month. After your belly begins to grow, avoid positions that have you lying face down. As with any exercise program, consult with your doctor before you begin.

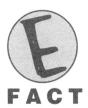

FACT

One of the essentials of yoga is breathing. In yoga you learn to breathe fully by taking in air slowly through the nose, filling your lungs entirely, and exhaling completely. Learning how to master this type of breathing can be twofold, helping you to prepare for labor and delivery.

When taking a yoga class, look for an instructor who is specially trained in prenatal yoga. Some yoga moves can be tricky, so if you feel pain or discomfort, make needed adjustments. Do not hold poses for too long, and move into and out of yoga positions slowly and carefully to avoid any injury or lightheadedness. As you become larger in your third trimester, use a chair or other sturdy prop for support to avoid losing your balance. Equipment such as blocks and straps can help you to more easily move through different poses with better stability. Avoid poses that are difficult and that you may not be familiar with as well as those that stretch the abdominal muscles too much. It is important to be extra careful because you are more prone to tearing and/or straining muscles and ligaments while pregnant.

Kegel Exercises

Kegel exercises can be very helpful once you get to the delivery room. Kegel or pelvic-floor muscle exercises are internal exercises that can be done to help strengthen the muscles that control your urethra, bladder, uterus, and rectum. This exercise strengthens the pelvic floor so that during delivery you are able to push more efficiently. Strengthening these muscles can also assist your body in recovering quicker after delivery. They can help with bladder control problems that many women experience after childbirth.

Kegels are done most simply by contracting and holding the muscles that are used to stop the flow of urine. Try to do Kegels in sets of ten, and work up to three to four sets about three times each day. Start out slow, and work your way up as these muscles become stronger. Make sure you are doing the exercises correctly. If you are not sure, ask your doctor.

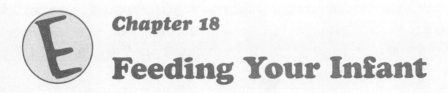

Chapter 18

Feeding Your Infant

Good nutrition for your little one right from the start will get him off to a healthy beginning. Breast milk or formula is the only food your infant needs for his first four to six months of life. If you decide to breastfeed, following some sound nutritional guidelines can ensure you are getting all of the calories and nutrients needed to nourish your baby properly.

Why Breastfeed?

One of the very first decisions new parents make is how to feed their newborn. Many health professionals agree that the ideal method is breastfeeding, though for some women this is not the best choice for physical, health, or personal reasons. For some mothers, breastfeeding is an easy transition. For others it may take some time and patience before the process is a smooth one. It is perfectly normal for it to take some time and practice. A lactation consultant should visit you in the hospital to help you get started.

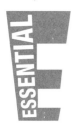

The American Dietetic Association (ADA) and the American Academy of Pediatrics (AAP) both recommend that babies be breastfed exclusively for the first four to six months of life and then breastfed with complementary foods for at least twelve months.

Benefits of Breastfeeding

Even though breastfeeding is not your only option, there are many benefits to using this method to nourish your newborn in the beginning. Breastfeeding can aid in the physical, emotional, and practical needs of both the baby and the mother. Other benefits include these:

- The infant is able to eat on demand without any trouble. When the infant is hungry, the milk is ready instantly without any measuring, mixing, or warming of bottles.
- There is no concern over proper sterilization.
- Breast milk is easy for babies to digest, so there is less spitting up.
- Breast milk is rich in antibodies that can help protect the baby from intestinal, ear, urinary, and lower respiratory-tract infections, as well as pneumonia.
- If breastfeeding is continued through at least the first six months of life, it can help decrease the risk of the baby's developing food allergies.
- In babies with a family history of food allergies, breastfeeding can help lower the risk of developing asthma and some skin conditions.

- The quality and the quantity of fat in breast milk tends to be more nutritious than the fat found in most formulas.
- Breastfeeding is less expensive than formula feeding.
- New studies indicate that breastfed infants may be less likely to become obese later in life and therefore less likely to develop diabetes.
- Women who breastfeed usually return to their pre-pregnancy weight more quickly, and the uterus also returns to its normal size more quickly.
- Breastfeeding can help reduce the risk of ovarian cancer and, in pre-menopausal women, breast cancer.

How the Body Produces Breast Milk

During pregnancy, the body naturally begins to prepare itself for breastfeeding. In the first few days after birth, a woman's body produces a fluid called colostrum. This is the first milk that the infant receives. Colostrum is a thick, yellowish substance that is produced just prior to the flow of breast milk. It contains antibodies and immunoglobulins, which help protect the newborn from bacteria and viruses and help to prevent the infant's immature gut from becoming infected. Colostrum is high in protein, zinc, and other minerals and contains less fat, carbohydrates, and calories than actual breast milk.

Between the third and sixth day after birth, colostrum begins to change to a "transitional" form of breast milk. During this time, the amounts of protein and immune factors in the milk gradually decrease while fat, lactose, and calories in the milk increase. By about the tenth day after birth, the mother begins to produce mature breast milk. One of the special qualities of breast milk is its ability to change to meet the needs of your growing baby throughout the course of breastfeeding.

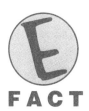

FACT

The size of breasts is not a factor in how much milk a mother produces. Instead it is the infant's feeding habits that control milk production. In other words, the more a woman breastfeeds her infant, the more milk her body will produce.

The Nutrition of Breast Milk

At this point, human breast milk provides the most optimal nutrition for infants. Breast milk seems to have the perfect balance of carbohydrates, fats, and proteins as well as vitamins and minerals that the infant needs. Breast milk contains just enough protein to keep from overloading the baby's immature kidneys. The protein in breast milk is mostly in the form of whey, which is what helps to make it easily digestible. The fat in breast milk is also easily absorbed by an infant's digestive system. Breast milk provides liberal amounts of vital essential fatty acids, saturated fats, triglycerides, and cholesterol. It contains long-chain polyunsaturated fatty acids that are essential for proper development of the central nervous system. Breast milk is relatively low in sodium and provides adequate amounts of minerals such as zinc, iron, and calcium, which reduce the demand for these nutrients from the mother.

Breast milk contains large amounts of lactose, or milk sugar. Lactose is utilized in the tissues of the brain and spinal cord and helps to provide the infant with energy. Breast milk contains only a small amount of iron, but the iron is in a form that is readily absorbed. Fifty percent of the iron in breast milk is absorbed, compared with only 4 to 10 percent of the iron in cow's milk or commercial infant formula.

The ABCs of Breastfeeding

Proper technique is important to make sure the process goes smoothly and the baby consumes enough milk. In addition to techniques, you will have plenty of questions as to how much, when, and how long. Take the time to get the advice, support, education, and encouragement you need from a lactation consultant, pediatrician, family, friends, and support groups.

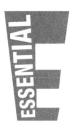

Breastfeeding requires much commitment from the mother. If you choose to go back to work outside of the home or if you are separated from your infant for other reasons, you can still breastfeed. In these cases, a breast pump can be used to collect breast milk when needed.

How Often to Breastfeed

If you have chosen to breastfeed, the process should begin as soon as possible after birth. Babies who are breastfed tend to feed more often than babies who are formula fed. Breastfed babies generally eat eight to twelve times per day. This is basically because breastfed babies' stomachs empty more quickly since breast milk is so easy to digest. The baby should eat until she is full, usually ten to fifteen minutes per breast. At first, most newborns want to eat every few hours, both during the day and at night. Babies generally eat on demand when they are hungry. However, to make sure your baby is eating enough in the beginning weeks, wake her up if she has not eaten in more than four hours. Look for signs from your baby that she is hungry, such as increased alertness or activity, mouthing, or rooting around the breast. Crying seems to be more of a later sign of hunger. As your baby gets older and becomes alert for longer periods of time, you can more easily settle into a routine schedule of feeding every three hours or so with fewer sessions at night. By the end of the first month, babies will generally start sleeping longer throughout the night.

Is My Baby Getting Enough Milk?

A worry for many breastfeeding moms is whether the newborn is getting enough to eat. With formulas, you are able to tell exactly how many ounces the baby has consumed, but with breastfeeding this is harder to identify. It may seem at first that the baby is hungry all the time, which makes some moms wonder if he has had enough. This is completely normal. Babies should be hungry quite often because breast milk is digested within a couple of hours after consumption. After the baby's first few days of life, he will want to nurse about eight to twelve times per day. The baby should be fed on demand, with no worry about schedules, until you have breastfeeding down pat and can begin to recognize your baby's own schedule. The baby's pediatrician will be able to tell if your baby is getting enough to eat by how much weight he gains at each visit.

There are other ways to tell if your baby is getting enough to eat. After the fifth day of birth, she should have at least six to eight wet diapers per day and three to four loose yellow stools per day. She is most likely getting enough if she is nursing at least ten to fifteen minutes on each breast. Your baby should show steady weight gain after the first week of age. Her urine should be pale yellow and not deep yellow or orange. You should find your baby wanting to eat at least every two to three hours or at least eight times per day for at least the first two to three weeks. In addition, she should have good skin color. If you become concerned about whether your baby is getting enough to eat, contact your pediatrician or lactation consultant. Babies who are not getting enough to eat can become easily dehydrated.

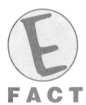

FACT

In general, most babies lose a little weight, 5 to 10 percent of their birth weight, in their first few days of life. They should start to gain at least 1 ounce per day by the fifth day after birth and be back to their birth weight by two weeks after birth.

Is Breast Milk Enough?

During the first six months of life, most babies who are breastfeeding will not require any additional water, juices, vitamins, iron, or formula. With sound breastfeeding practices, supplements are rarely needed because breast milk provides the infant with just about all the fluids and nutrients he needs for proper growth and development. By six months of age, it is generally recommended that babies be introduced to foods that contain iron in addition to breast milk.

While the water supply in most U.S. cities and towns contains plenty of fluoride, a mineral often found in tap water that is important for strong teeth and prevention of cavities, in certain rural areas the levels can be too low. Breast milk contains very low levels of fluoride. However, babies under six months of age should not be given fluoride supplements, even if levels in your water supply are low.

Vitamin D Controversy

Though breast milk is a complete source of nutrition for your baby, there is some controversy surrounding the need for supplementing with vitamin D. Vitamin D is found in only small amounts in breast milk and is necessary to absorb calcium into the bones and teeth. However, the vitamin D in breast milk is in a very absorbable form and therefore is generally adequate for most infants. Babies who may be at higher risk for vitamin D deficiency include those who have little exposure to sunlight. Moderate sunlight helps to produce vitamin D in the body, and mother and babies with darker skin may have a harder time getting enough sunlight to produce vitamin D.

Mothers deficient in vitamin D also create a risk of low levels in their babies. The amount of vitamin D in breast milk is directly related to the level of vitamin D in the mother's body. If you are taking a prenatal or vitamin/mineral supplement that contains vitamin D, drinking milk, and getting moderate exposure to sunlight, your breast milk should contain optimal levels of vitamin D. The American Academy of Pediatrics recently began recommending that all infants, including those who are exclusively breastfed, have a minimum intake of 200 international units (IU) of vitamin D per day beginning in the first two months of life.

Other Concerns

Babies sometimes react to certain foods that the mother eats because they may pass through to the breast milk. After eating spicy or gassy foods, the mother may notice the baby crying or fussing as well as nursing more often. However, these symptoms may also show up in babies with colic. You will know it is a reaction to food you have eaten if the symptoms last less than twenty-four hours. Symptoms caused by colic generally occur daily and often last for days or weeks at a time. If your baby seems to react to certain foods that you eat, eliminate those foods from your diet. There is no need to eliminate foods from your diet unless you have a specific reason to suspect a particular food is bothering your baby. If you have a family history of allergies, including asthma, you may want to avoid foods you are allergic or sensitive to while breastfeeding.

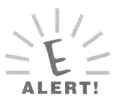
ALERT!

The American Academy of Pediatrics suggests that breastfeeding mothers of susceptible infants (with a family history of allergies) are wise to eliminate peanuts and peanut-containing foods while breastfeeding.

Although the reaction is rare, some babies are allergic to cow's milk and foods that contain cow's milk in the mother's diet. Symptoms will usually appear a few minutes to a few hours after a breastfeeding session. They can include diarrhea, rash, fussiness, gas, runny nose, cough, or congestion. Talk to your pediatrician if your baby experiences any of these symptoms. Other foods you consume that may cause reactions in your newborn include chocolate, citrus fruits and juices, and common food allergens such as eggs, wheat, corn, fish, nuts, and soy.

Nutritional Requirements for the Breastfeeding Mom

As with pregnancy, it is vital that a mother eat a healthy, well-balanced diet to ensure that she gets all of the nutrients she needs for successful breastfeeding. The mother's diet needs to fulfill her own nutritional needs as well as additional needs, which increase during breastfeeding. At this time your body's first priority is milk production, and if you lack the right type of nourishment in your diet, your personal needs may not be met.

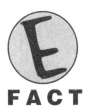

FACT

Women who were obese prior to pregnancy or who gained excessive weight during pregnancy may not require the full 500 extra calories per day. Your doctor can help to calculate the amount of additional calories you may need during breastfeeding.

Calorie Needs

Your body's fuel supply for milk production comes from two main sources: extra calories, or energy, from foods you eat and energy stored as body fat during pregnancy. For your body to produce breast milk, it uses about 100 to 150 calories a day from fat that your body naturally stored during pregnancy. That is why breastfeeding moms often lose pregnancy weight more quickly. In addition, you also need to eat about 500 extra calories per day (or 500 calories more than your maintenance calorie level) during breastfeeding. In general, consuming 500 extra calories per day than before pregnancy will meet your energy needs for breast milk production.

Figuring on light to moderate activity, on average a woman needs about 2,700 calories per day. You need more calories if you are a teenager or more active. You can easily get these extra calories by eating nutritious foods from all of the food groups in the Food Guide Pyramid. The following number of servings from the Food Guide Pyramid would provide about 2,700 calories:

- 10 servings from the bread, cereal, rice, and pasta group (choose whole grains and whole-wheat products more often)
- 4 servings from the vegetable group
- 4 servings from the fruit group
- 3–4 servings of dairy (choose nonfat or low-fat dairy products). Teens should shoot for 4 servings per day
- 2 servings (6–7 ounces) from the meat, poultry, fish, dry beans, eggs, and nut group (choose leaner meats more often as well as occasionally choose nonmeat selections such as legumes, nuts, or seeds)
- Use fats and sweets sparingly

Once breastfeeding is well established, a mother can reduce the number of excess calories modestly. This will increase the rate the body uses stored fat without an adverse impact on breast-milk production. Be cautious not to cut calories drastically during breastfeeding, which can reduce daily milk production.

How to Fuel Your Body

While you are breastfeeding, it is still important to remember that you are still eating for two. You need to continue the healthy diet you followed during pregnancy through breastfeeding and beyond. Not only is it important to get extra calories, but those extra calories need to come from healthy foods. Eating a healthy, well-balanced diet will ensure you are getting the carbohydrates, protein, and healthy fats you need for breastfeeding. Focus on fueling your body with whole-grain starches, fresh fruits and vegetables, and lean protein foods that will provide plenty of protein, calcium, and iron.

Simply adding empty calories to increase your caloric intake, such as with sugary or high-fat foods, is not going to be advantageous to you or your baby. Eating a variety of foods is important because this way, you can be sure to obtain different nutrients. Eating in moderation is the key, not too much of any one food or item.

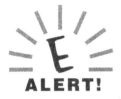

ALERT!

Rapid weight loss and cutting calories too low can pose a danger to your baby. Since milk production requires extra calorie expenditure, even increasing your caloric level by 500 calories will allow for a safe amount of weight loss. Losing weight gradually through a healthy, well-balanced diet and regular exercise is the safest route.

Nutrient Needs of the Breastfeeding Mom

The process of breastfeeding is nutritionally demanding for a mother. During breastfeeding your need for many nutrients will increase even more than during pregnancy. The amount of milk you produce is not likely affected by the food you consume, unless you cut your calories drastically. However, the composition of your milk may vary with certain nutrients depending on your dietary intake.

Calcium

Though your calcium needs don't change during breastfeeding, calcium is still an important nutrient during this time. The recommended amount of 1,000 mg for women over nineteen is a must. If you come up short, your body may draw from the calcium reserves in your bones, which can put you at greater risk for osteoporosis later in life. It can also cause periodontal problems down the line. In addition to dairy foods, choose other foods high in calcium such as dark-green leafy vegetables, fish with edible bones, almonds, and fortified beverages.

B Vitamins

A few of the B vitamins deserve special mention, including vitamin B_{12}, folic acid, and vitamin B_6. The daily recommended intake for vitamin B_{12} increases slightly during breastfeeding. If you are a strict vegetarian, your breast milk might be missing adequate stores of vitamin B_{12}. Ensure your prenatal or multivitamin contains adequate amounts of vitamin B_{12}. If you are not a vegetarian, you most likely are getting enough. Folic acid, another B vitamin, is important especially if you are considering another pregnancy soon. Vitamin B_6 increases slightly during breastfeeding, and women often do not consume enough. Chicken, fish, and pork are great sources of this B vitamin as well as whole-grain products and legumes.

Iron

Iron requirements are lower after your baby is born and you are breast-feeding. The needs go down to 9 mg per day for adult women until you begin to menstruate again, in which case needs go back to normal (18 mg per day). If you are taking an iron supplement, it will not increase iron levels in your breast milk. Anemia in nursing moms has been associated with decreased milk supply. If you are anemic, you should speak to your doctor about a safe dosage of iron supplementation. You can often improve your condition by making changes to your diet. Including foods with absorbable iron sources and including a source of vitamin C with these foods can help to bring up your iron levels.

Zinc

Zinc requirements only increase slightly from pregnancy to breastfeeding. You lose some zinc when breastfeeding, and your diet may not always be able to compensate for the loss. If you are taking a prenatal or multivitamin, it should take care of any zinc requirements you may not be getting.

Supplements During Breastfeeding

Some doctors may recommend continuing your prenatal supplement through breastfeeding. You can get enough nutrients through the foods you eat if you consistently make good choices. If you come up short on your calories or nutrients, your breast milk is usually still sufficient for supporting your baby's proper growth and development. Unless you are severely malnourished, your breast milk will provide what the infant requires. However, this will be at the expense of your own nutrient reserves. Keep in mind that vitamin and mineral supplements should never be used to make up for poor eating habits.

Essential Fluids

You need to drink lots of fluids and stay well hydrated while breastfeeding. A hormone called oxytocin that is released by your body during breastfeeding tends to make you thirsty. Although fluids will not directly affect your milk supply, it is still recommended to drink at least eight to twelve glasses of water each day.

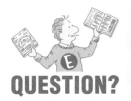

QUESTION?

Can I exercise while I am breastfeeding?
It is safe to exercise at a moderate level after breastfeeding is well established. Aerobic exercise at 60 to 70 percent of your maximal heart rate seems to be safe and has no adverse affects on breastfeeding or milk production. However, strenuous exercise that results in lactic acid production may cause breast milk to taste sour to babies. This can happen up to ninety minutes after exercise, so plan breastfeeding sessions accordingly. Also keep in mind that you may need more calories and more fluids according to your level and frequency of exercise.

Harmful Substances

As with pregnancy, is it essential to think about all the substances you put into your body that can pass through to your breast milk and on to your baby. Many medications are safe to take during breastfeeding, but a few, including herbal products and/or supplements, can be dangerous to your infant. Always get approval from your doctor before taking any prescription or over-the-counter medications while breastfeeding. Alcohol should be avoided because it can pass through your breast milk to the baby. You would be wise to cut back on caffeine due to the fact that it can build up in a baby's system. A cup or two a day of coffee or cola is not likely to do harm, but too much can lead to problems. The guidelines for eating fish (due to mercury levels, as discussed in Chapter 7) also pertain to women who are breastfeeding. Habits such as smoking and illegal drugs can cause a mother to produce less milk, and chemicals such as nicotine can pass through the breast milk.

Formula Feeding

Don't beat yourself up if you cannot breastfeed for some reason. Many women cannot breastfeed for medical, physical, or other reasons. If you are not able to breastfeed or choose not to, today's infant formulas do provide a good nutritious alternative. Most are manufactured in a way that closely mimics, as much as possible, the components of breast milk. They are made to be easy for babies to digest and provide all of the nutrition needed. It is virtually impossible for a mother to create a formula at home that would have the same complex combination of proteins, sugars, fats, vitamins, and minerals that a baby needs and that are present in commercial formulas and breast milk. Therefore, if you do not breastfeed your baby, you should use only a commercially prepared formula.

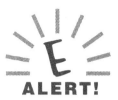

ALERT!

Because of its contents, cow's milk is not appropriate for infants younger than twelve months. Although some formulas are cow-milk based, they have been modified to meet an infant's special needs.

What's in Formula?

Commercial formulas are usually cow-milk based and are fortified with iron as well as other essential vitamins and minerals. Some manufactures even include some substances found directly in breast milk that can be manufactured. For infants who cannot tolerate cow's milk, there are also soy-based formulas. Formula feeding is more costly than breastfeeding but, on the other hand, is more convenient for some mothers. Today's commercial formula products are manufactured under strict sterile conditions, so there is no worry about contamination.

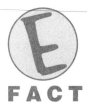

FACT

Iron-fortified infant formulas have been credited for the declining incidence of iron deficiency anemia in infants. For this reason, the American Academy of Pediatrics highly recommends that mothers who are not breastfeeding use an iron-fortified infant formula.

The Pros and Cons

Some women feel that formula-feeding their infant gives them a little more freedom and that other members of the family, such as the father, can be more active in the feeding and caring of the infant. Just as breastfeeding has its own unique demands, so does formula feeding. The main demands of formula feeding are organization, handling, and proper preparation. You need to make sure to have enough formula on hand, and bottles must be prepared very carefully using sterile methods. The bottles and nipples must be kept sanitary and ready for when you need them.

Preparing Formulas

Commercial formulas come in all types of varieties. There are ready-to-feed liquids, concentrated liquids that require diluting with water, and powders that require mixing with water. You should always follow closely the instructions on the label for preparing bottles. As well as varieties of formulas, there are many different types of bottles and nipples available to choose from. You may need to experiment with a few different brands before you find a combination that works best for you and your baby.

Bottles should be warmed just slightly before feeding. Never heat a bottle of formula in a microwave! The formula can heat unevenly and leave hot spots, which can burn a baby's mouth. A microwave can also heat the formula too much, making it too hot for an infant's mouth. The best way is to heat water in the microwave, take the water out, and then heat the bottle in the water. Always test the formula to make sure the temperature is not too hot. Always wash bottles and nipples thoroughly in hot water, and wash your hands before preparing them.

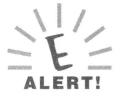

ALERT!

Do not leave bottles out of the refrigerator for longer than one hour. If your baby doesn't finish a bottle, the contents should be discarded. If formula bottles are prepared in advance, they should be stored in the refrigerator for no longer than twenty-four hours.

How Often to Formula Feed

Experts agree that for the first few weeks, you shouldn't try to follow too rigid a feeding schedule. As the baby gets older, you may be able to work out a more established schedule. You should offer a bottle every two to three hours at first as you see signs of hunger. Until she reaches about 10 pounds, she will probably take approximately two to 3 ounces per feeding. From there, intake will gradually increase. Don't force her to eat if she does not seem hungry. You may see certain signs when the baby has enough such as, closing her mouth or turning away from the bottle, falling asleep, fussiness, and biting or playing with the bottle's nipple. One advantage to bottle feeding is that you can know exactly how much your baby is eating. You pediatrician can advise you on optimal amounts to feed your baby as she grows.

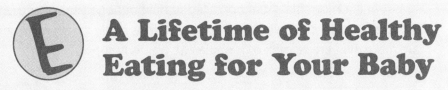

Chapter 19

A Lifetime of Healthy Eating for Your Baby

By following sound and realistic nutrition guidelines, you can help get your new baby off to a lifetime of healthy eating. The key is providing your child with a diet full of good nutrition and healthy calories to support her proper growth and development. Starting young will help teach your child good habits that she can carry throughout her life. Feeding your child can be frustrating, so be patient and use plenty of creativity. Make mealtimes fun!

Starting Baby on Solid Foods

When you start your baby on solid foods, you begin lifelong eating habits that will contribute to his overall health throughout life. The American Academy of Pediatrics recommends feeding your child only breast milk or formula for the first four to six months of life. After that, a combination of solid food and breast milk or formula should be used until about one year of age. After six months of age, your newborn's nutritional needs begin to increase, until they are more than breast milk or formula can properly supply.

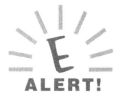

ALERT!

Do not start solid foods too early in your child's diet. The intestinal tract and immune systems are not yet fully developed, so introducing solid foods too early can cause babies to develop food allergies. The other danger of feeding too early is a baby's inability to chew or swallow properly before four to six months of age.

When and How to Start

Even though you may choose to breastfeed past four to six months, at this age your baby should be ready to add some solid foods. By this age babies need more calories and iron than breast milk or formula alone can supply. Although most babies are generally ready to start solid foods between four and six months, this is only a point of reference. All babies are different, and they need to be ready both physically and developmentally to start on solid foods. Offering your baby solids too early can lead to some frustrating feeding times for both the parents and the infant. The following may be clues that your baby is ready:

- Your baby weighs at least 13 pounds and has doubled his birth weight.
- Your baby can sit with a little support as well as somewhat control his head.
- Your baby seems to still be hungry after eight to ten feedings of breast milk, or he can drink more than 32 ounces of formula a day.

- Your baby seems to show some interest in foods that you are eating.
- Your baby can move foods from the front to the back of his mouth. When younger than four months or not ready, babies will push foods out of their mouths with their tongues. As they develop, the tongue becomes more coordinated and can move back and forth, which helps babies to eat from a spoon.

Never force your baby to start solids. If you try and she does not seem interested, wait a few weeks and try again. Remember that all babies are different and will begin at their own pace.

The Four- to Six-Month Period

The solid food most recommended for feeding your child in the beginning is an iron-fortified rice cereal. Your baby's first cereal feeding should be a thin mixture. Start by mixing about one tablespoon of rice cereal with breast milk or formula (usually one part cereal to four parts liquid). Read the suggested mixing directions on the box for the product you choose, and do not add anything extra such as sugar or honey.

Use a baby-feeding spoon with a rubber tip or simply your finger to feed. Start by offering the cereal mixture once a day, and as your baby tolerates it, increase to two to three times a day. Keep in mind that she probably won't eat too much at one time. Her tummy is small and can only tolerate small portions. Most of her nutrition will still come from breast milk or formula at this point. As your baby begins to become used to have semisolid food in her mouth, you can add a little less liquid to make it a bit thicker. This will help her to work on chewing and swallowing.

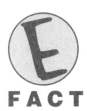

FACT

After your baby has eaten rice cereal for several days with no signs of intolerance or allergies, you can offer barley or oat cereal if you choose. However, do not offer wheat cereal until after twelve months of age because some infants are sensitive or allergic to wheat before this age.

At about five to six months, after cereal has passed the test, you can start to offer single pureed or strained fruits and vegetables in addition to breast milk or formula and iron-fortified cereal. It may be beneficial to start with vegetables because once your baby learns to like the sweet taste of fruit, you may have a hard time getting him to eat vegetables. Good fruits and vegetables to start with include sweet potatoes, squash, applesauce, bananas, carrots, peaches, and pears. All foods at this point should be mushy or strained. As your baby is offered more foods, he will take less breast milk or formula. However, these feeding should still be continued and should remain the mainstay of his diet for the first year.

Introduce only one new food at a time over a three- to five-day period when starting your baby on solid foods. This will help rule out food allergies and intolerances. Once you introduce a food and you are sure your baby tolerates it with no adverse reaction such as skin rashes, wheezing, diarrhea, or stomachaches, move on to another new food. As your baby gets older and is introduced to a wider variety of foods, keep an eye on highly allergenic foods such as wheat, egg whites, cow's milk, peanuts, fish, soy, and dairy foods.

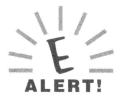

ALERT!

Children under twelve months of age should avoid eating honey because it can cause infant botulism.

The Six- to Nine-Month Period

By six months of age, your baby's digestive tract is more mature, and she has mastered the art of chewing and swallowing. At this stage you can begin introducing all kinds of strained and mashed food along with the standard breast milk or formula and iron-fortified cereal. In addition to fruits and vegetables, you can try other strained or puréed foods such as plain meats and poultry, egg yolks (continue to avoid egg whites), sweet potatoes, squash, mashed beans, and unsweetened fruit juices (vitamin C–fortified) such as apple or pear in a sippy cup (not a bottle). As her feeding skills increase and she gets more teeth, she can move on to minced and finely chopped foods and soft foods. Avoid combination meat-and-vegetable dinners at this time.

Around seven months, your baby will want to begin feeding himself. Nature will take its course—let him begin with foods such as unsweetened dry cereal, dry toast, crackers, or teething biscuits. Between six and nine months, most babies will become interested in drinking from a cup. You can offer juice, water, or formula at this time in a child spill-proof cup. Juice is not necessary but can provide a little variety.

Nine to Twelve Months

Between nine and twelve months, your baby will be even more interested in feeding herself and be ready for soft table foods as well as a wider variety of finger foods. Keep in mind that you should still be feeding breast milk or formula along with these foods. By the end of the first year, solid food will make up about 50 percent of your baby's intake.

Begin with soft, bite-sized pieces of food that she can pick up and eat such as cooked vegetables, mashed potatoes, ripened soft fruit without peels or seeds, soft breads, lean tender meats, and noodles. You can also begin using junior jar foods. As her breast milk and formula intake begins to decrease, you can offer yogurt, cheese, and cottage cheese. Increase the amount of food you are feeding your baby according to her appetite. It is important to offer a variety of foods to encourage good eating habits later in life.

Foods to Avoid

During the first year, avoid giving your child foods that may be difficult to chew or swallow or that could be a choking hazard. This can include large pieces of meat or poultry, hot dogs, nuts, seeds, popcorn, pretzels, raisins, raw carrots, grapes, and hard candy. Chop these foods up into small pieces before serving to your child.

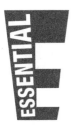

Peanut butter should not be offered until after age three due to possible allergic reactions, especially if either parent has an allergy to peanuts.

Avoid giving your child chewing gum. Always watch your baby or be in the room as he eats in case of choking. This includes watching older brothers or sisters who can give your baby food he is not ready for.

Wait until your child is older than twelve months to start offering cow's milk. Most experts recommend whole milk over any lower-fat variety until your child is older than two. If using soy milk after twelve months of age, be sure it is whole soy milk and not the low-fat or nonfat versions. Fat is important for brain development in children under two. In addition, be sure the soy milk is fortified with vitamin A, vitamin D, and calcium.

Your Growing Kid: The Early Years

Once your child reaches the age of two, his diet will basically consist of solid foods. At this age, children really begin to master the skill of eating, and they are curious about trying new foods. This is the time, when they are very impressionable, to help them start good lifelong eating habits. Undoubtedly, you will have questions and concerns about whether your child is eating nutritionally adequate amount and types of food. Though every child has unique needs as well as preferences, you can follow some general guidelines to ensure your child is getting all he needs.

Energy Needs

Once your child reaches toddler and preschool age, her growth rate will start to slow down. Basically, she needs enough energy or calories to fuel her activity and her various growth spurts. At this age, she does not yet need adult-sized portions. In fact, feeding her large portions can overwhelm her small appetites and can be too much for her small stomach.

The American Academy of Pediatrics recommends that children age one to three get approximately forty calories for every inch of height. For example, if your toddler is thirty inches tall, he should get about 1,300 calories per day for normal growth and weight gain. Keep in mind this is only an estimate. Calorie needs will vary greatly from child to child depending on their activity level as well as their metabolism. Most kids eat when they are hungry and stop when they are full. They generally get what their bodies need as long as you offer them a healthy variety of foods at regular meal and snack times. Do not force your child to eat. Instead, let her appetite guide her food intake. If you worry about your child getting too little or too much food, speak to your child's pediatrician.

Food Guide Pyramid for Young Children

Your child's calorie intake should come from a daily variety of grains, vegetables, fruits, dairy, and protein foods such as lean meats. Carbohydrates should make up much of their energy needs. They also need plenty of protein and moderate amounts of fat for proper growth and development as well as to meet their energy needs. Since children have limited stomach capacity, feeding them five to six small meals per day will work best. To make sure your child is eating enough use the Food Guide Pyramid for Young Children (two to six years old) as a general guide for planning daily meals and snacks, as follows:

- 6 servings of grains including breads, cereal, rice, pasta, and crackers
- 3 servings of vegetables, including fresh and cooked
- 2 servings of fruit including fresh, cooked, canned, or 100-percent juice drinks
- 2 servings of protein foods including meat, fish, poultry, tofu, beans, peas, and lentils
- 2 servings of low-fat dairy products including milk, cheese, and yogurt
- Fats and sweets should be consumed in moderation

It is fine for children to eat higher-fat foods such as chicken fingers, French fries, ice cream, and all the other foods they will mostly likely choose, on occasion. Just make sure that healthier foods are also offered and consumed along with these foods. Keep in mind that a child's appetite can be very unpredictable, changing from day to day and with sporadic growth spurts. Be patient and prepared—your child may refuse meals one day and ask for seconds the next. Again, children are great judges as to how much they need and want to eat. As long as they are growing normally, they are probably getting enough calories.

Fighting Food Jags

Food jags are the periods when your child refuses foods that he previously liked or when he requests a particular food over and over again. Food jags are very common in toddlers and preschoolers between two and six years of age. It's a habit that can be extremely frustrating, and it causes concern for many parents. Food jags can happen for many reasons, including boredom with the usual foods, an especial interest in familiar foods, or a means of discovering new independence.

The best way to handle food jags is to remain calm and remember that they are temporary. The more you dwell on the problem food, the longer the food jag may last. Don't force your child to eat something he doesn't want or take away a food he keeps asking for. Instead of forcing your child to eat something he does not want, don't offer it for a while and bring it back down the line. If he wants the same food constantly, give it to him, but include other foods with it for variety and nutritional intake. Most children will become bored with foods after awhile and move on to something new.

You can also include your child in choosing foods at the grocery store and/or preparing foods at home to help them expand their choices. Most importantly, don't worry. Children will generally meet all of their nutritional needs over several days' time. If your child tends to refuse entire food groups over several weeks, speak to your pediatrician or dietitian so you can substitute foods and possibly start a child's vitamin/mineral supplement that will ensure adequate nutritional intake.

Introducing New Foods

Variety in a child's diet is important for good nutritional intake, yet it can be more than frustrating to get your child to try new foods. In addition to taste, many factors are important to a child's acceptance of new foods. The temperature, odor, and presentation of food are also important in whether a child will be open to trying a new food. To help your child try new foods, offer just one new food at a time to keep things from being overwhelming. Let your child know ahead of time if the new food will taste sweet, sour or salty so she is not surprised, and just give a very small amount to taste at first to see if she likes it. Keep in mind that most children do best with foods that are lukewarm in temperature.

Take the time to explain that you just want him to taste the new food, and if he doesn't like it, he doesn't have to swallow it. To urge him to try something new, sit the child with a sibling or friend who is a good taster and can be counted on to eat the food. Monkey see, monkey do! Serving a new food with a food that the child already likes and is familiar with can help him feel more comfortable about trying something new. Present the food in a fun way, and be creative. Most important, if your child doesn't accept the food the first time, don't give up! Try it again later down the road.

The best way to get your child to try new foods, eat a healthy diet, eat vegetables, and drink her milk every day is if you—her parents—do also. Be a good role model, and teach your child through taking action. Actions speak much louder than words, and the better you do, the better she will do. Going easy on higher-fat, higher-calorie, higher-sugar food is good advice for the entire family. Family meals and snacks that are prepared with less fat and more healthy foods teach children good eating habits for a lifetime.

The Overweight Child

Are you beginning to wonder or worry that your youngster may be overweight? Even though some overweight infants grow up to be overweight children—and possibly adults—many also do not. It is difficult to tell if a child is overweight because kids grow at different rates and go through numerous growth spurts. Let your pediatrician be the judge of whether your child is in the healthy range. The doctor will use growth charts to measure your child's height and weight to make a proper determination.

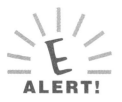

ALERT!

Never assume that because your child looks overweight, he must have a weight problem. Never restrict your child's diet to help him lose weight. Drastically limiting what a child eats can be harmful to his health and can interfere with proper growth and development. If you feel there is a problem, take your child to his pediatrician before taking any type of action.

What to Do

Children become overweight for a variety of reasons. The most common are genetic factors, lack of physical activity, unhealthy eating patterns, or a combination of any of these factors. In rare cases, a medical problem can cause a child to become overweight.

If your doctor feels there is a problem, you may need to make some changes in your child's food habits. It is more important to help your child adopt healthy eating and exercise habits than to count pounds lost.

To help your child achieve a healthier weight, try the following:

- Ensure your child is eating a well-balanced diet with plenty of fruits and vegetables and not eating too many empty calories or junk foods.
- After your child reaches the age of two, use fat-free or low-fat milk as opposed to whole milk.
- Make sure you child has plenty of opportunity to be physically active.
- Seek the advice of a health-care professional, such as a registered dietitian, to learn what and how much your child should be eating.
- Refrain from rewarding your child for good behavior with food such as ice cream or fast food.
- Keep in mind that adult approaches to weight loss are not fit for children.
- Support your child and encourage her, no matter what her weight.
- Start early in childhood, teaching your child good nutrition habits, selection of healthy low-fat snacks, and the importance of physical activity.
- Monitor the time your child spends watching television or sitting at a computer.
- Make it a point to include good nutrition and exercise as a family affair. Plan lower-fat meals for the entire family, have more nutritious snacks in the house, and plan fun family activities.
- Beware of using food as a reward for a certain accomplishment, as a substitute for affection, or as a compensation for a disappointment. Use other avenues as rewards.
- Make sure your child's portions are a child's size as opposed to an adult's. Use smaller plates for children so you and your child are not tempted to fill up a large adult--size plate.

- Stock your kitchen with low-fat and low-calorie snack foods that are quickly available when your child is hungry and grabbing something to eat. Eliminate most high-fat, high-calorie foods from the house.
- Instead of indulging in heavy snacking, make meals your child's primary source of calories.
- Do not force your child to clean her plate or to continue eating when she voices that she is full.
- Avoid labeling foods as "good" or "bad" and telling her she cannot have certain foods. Instead, teach your child how to fit all types of food into a healthy eating pattern and teach her how to eat in moderation.
- Make a family rule that eating is only allowed in the kitchen or dining room to keep kids from constantly snacking on high-calorie foods while watching television.

Growth Charts

At regular visits, your pediatrician will use growth charts to monitor your child's growth rate. By plotting a child's height and weight measurements on these charts, doctors are able to compare growth patterns with data collected on thousands of other U.S. children. This helps to determine whether a child's growth is normal compared with others of the same age. Boys and girls need to be plotted on different charts because of the difference in their growth rates and patterns. There are two sets of standard charts for both boys and girls: one for infants up to thirty-six months and another for children ages two to twenty years. The charts are a series of percentile curves that show the distribution of growth measurements of children from across the country.

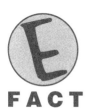

FACT

Older children are measured for height for age, weight for age, weight for height and—a recent addition—body mass index (BMI). An infant usually is measured for length for age, weight for age, weight for length, and head circumference for age.

A growth chart contains seven curves that all follow the same pattern. Each curve represents a different percentile: 5th, 10th, 25th, 50th, 75th, 90th, and 95th. The 50th percentile line represents an average value for the child's age. If, for example, a child's head circumference puts him in the 90th percentile, this means that his measurement is greater than or equal to the measurements of 90 percent of children in the country in his age category. The remaining 10 percent of children that age have head measurements that are bigger.

Just because a child has a high or low measurement at one visit does not necessarily mean there is a problem. Growth charts can be valuable tools. However, it is important not to focus too much on any one measure. Growth charts mean more when they are examined over a period of time. They then reveal a pattern of development. It is the pattern that tells you whether a child is growing properly in relation to other children of the same age and also shows how the child is progressing from measurement to measurement. Ask your doctor to share your child's growth chart progression with you at regular visits.

Finding Out About Food Allergies

An estimated 4 to 6 percent of infants and 1 to 2 percent of children are diagnosed with true food allergies. The most common food allergies in children include milk, eggs, peanuts, soybeans, tree nuts, wheat, fish, and shellfish. Children are likely to grow out of allergies to milk and soy by the time they are about three years old. Food allergies to peanuts, fish, shellfish, wheat, and eggs are seldom outgrown. Anyone can develop food allergies, but those with a family history are at higher risk. A true food allergy sets off a chain of immune system reactions when the offending food is consumed. When a child eats a food she is allergic to, her body releases antibodies that cause reactions such as skin rashes, runny nose, watery eyes, nausea, wheezing, or diarrhea. In rare cases, food allergies can cause anaphylactic shock, a much more severe reaction. Some food allergies symptoms in children show up immediately, while others may take a few days.

Food allergies are different than food sensitivities. Food sensitivity refers to an oral sensitivity that a child may experience when eating a specific food. The food may cause tingling, burning, itching, or other discomfort in the mouth or on the lips. It can progress to swelling in the mouth or throat, much like other serious allergic reactions. If your child experiences these types of symptoms, avoid the food and speak to your doctor.

If your child is at a high risk of developing food allergies, you should not offer solid foods until he is at least six months old. Once your child begins solid foods, avoid egg whites, cow's milk, and wheat until your infant it at least one year old. To be on the safe side also avoid peanuts (including peanut butter) until your child is at least three, especially if either parent has a history of a peanut allergy. Be careful of feeding your child mixed-ingredient foods or mixed entrees, such as casseroles, unless you are sure that he is not allergic to any of the individual ingredients. These types of food also make it difficult to determine food allergies. You should avoid adding any seasonings to your child's food until he is a bit older. Introduce new foods every three to five days—if your child is going to have an allergic reaction to a food, symptoms will either show up immediately or within this time frame.

If you suspect an allergic reaction to a certain food, keep a food diary for a few weeks and record what foods your child has been eating, especially recently introduced foods, and when he developed symptoms. Speak to your pediatrician, who may refer you to an allergist to ensure it is a true food allergy. An allergist may do some testing to determine the exact allergy. Avoiding a particular food in your child's diet can sometimes be more difficult than it sounds. Foods can show up as ingredients in other foods, and depending on the severity of the allergy, a little bit may be enough to trigger a severe reaction.

It is essential to learn all you can about your child's specific food allergy. A registered dietitian can help. Your doctor should be the one to let you know when it might be safe to reintroduce the food. If your child experiences more severe symptoms, speak with your pediatrician immediately.

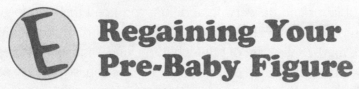

Chapter 20

Regaining Your Pre-Baby Figure

It can be both exciting and overwhelming to start thinking of regaining your pre-baby figure and getting into your favorite pair of jeans again. Keep in mind that it took almost nine months to put that pregnancy weight on—it will take some time to take it off. Most important, be patient and take a sensible approach to weight loss.

When Is It Safe to Start Losing the Weight?

Even though you are probably very eager to get started on weight loss after the birth of your baby, you should generally wait at least six weeks before beginning. This applies to women who breastfeed as well as to those who don't. You need to give your body some time to recover from the physical demands of labor and delivery. In addition, you need the time to get your life back in order: deal with the needs of your newborn, help manage your household, maybe take care of other children, and—for some—prepare to return to work. Most women do this on a lot less sleep, so go easy on yourself and give yourself a little time to get situated. Your doctor should be the one to give you the go-ahead to start slimming down or to exercising after delivery. This time frame will depend on many factors, such as whether you had a vaginal or cesarean delivery, whether you experienced any complications during pregnancy such as preeclampsia or gestational diabetes, and whether you were in good shape before your pregnancy.

For some women, pregnancy causes permanent changes in body shape, including slightly wider hips or waistline. The good news is that the majority of women lose a significant portion of the weight they gained during pregnancy within the first month of delivery. The bad news is that the weight left over is much slower and harder to get off. So be patient! It can take up to a year to lose the remaining weight and get back your muscle tone. Of course, all women differ. This time frame depends on many factors, including your pre-pregnancy weight and fitness level, your determination to lose the weight, your age, and your lifestyle.

Smart Weight Loss

It is important to be patient and take a sensible approach to weight loss. Generally, a sensible approach includes increasing physical activity and moderately decreasing the amount of healthy calories you eat by watching your portion sizes. For women who are breastfeeding, calorie intake should not be decreased until they are done breastfeeding. Don't let this frustrate you, though. In general, breastfeeding women tend to lose weight naturally, even with additional calories, because their bodies are burning calories simply through the process of breastfeeding. Breastfeeding requires about 800 calories daily. Stored body fat from pregnancy kicks in about 300 calories for milk production. Your dietary intake needs to supply the rest. That adds up to about an extra 500 calories per day, or 200 more calories than you needed during pregnancy.

You may not be advised to diet, but you can still eat a healthy diet, avoid empty calories, and exercise with your doctor's permission. An 8-ounce to 2-pound weight loss per week (1 pound if you're breastfeeding) is considered healthy. Rapid weight loss can affect breastfeeding and comes from a loss of fluid and muscle—your goal, on the other hand, is to lose fat.

A Healthy Plan

A healthy weight loss plan does not need to be complicated or expensive. If you were eating a healthy diet during pregnancy, then you simply continue those habits while eating less. You need to devise a healthy eating plan that includes plenty of fruits, vegetables, and whole grains. Include fat-free or low-fat dairy products and lean proteins such as lean meats, poultry, fish, legumes, and soy as well. Your best bet is to visit a registered dietitian who can give you the education and guidance you need to lose weight safely and effectively as well as keep it off for a lifetime.

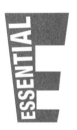

One of the biggest problem areas for women after pregnancy is the belly. Abdominal muscles stretched during pregnancy usually become loose in the period after childbirth and give you the "pouch" look. The only way to get rid of excess body fat is to burn more energy than you are taking in.

Losing Tips

Follow some simple guidelines to lose weight the smart way. Become physically active by walking, or take up another aerobic activity for thirty minutes a day most days of the week. Check with your doctor before starting to exercise. Stick to a healthy plan that provides about 1,200 to 1,500 calories per day. This level depends on many factors including your amount of physical activity as well as your age. If you are breastfeeding, you will need calories. Keep your fat intake to no more than 30 percent of your total calories (30 percent is about 40 grams of fat on a 1,200 calorie diet). When watching your fat intake, fat-free and lower-fat products are a better choice. However, don't forget that these foods still contain calories and that you do need some healthy fats in your diet.

Include at least five servings of fruit and vegetables in your diet each day. In addition to the health benefits of a plant-based diet, the fiber in fruits and vegetables will help you feel full and help you eat less. Drinking all of your recommended water each day can also act as an appetite buffer. Plan your meals ahead of time; thinking ahead can really help you choose healthy foods and cut back on the total calories you eat. Eating breakfast every day can help you manage your weight and may help curb binge eating later in the day.

Changing your eating habits can be tough—expect temptation, and have a plan of alternative strategies already mapped out. Try keeping a food journal of what and when you eat. People who lose weight gradually (½ to 2 pounds per week) are more likely to keep the weight off. Weigh yourself once a week to monitor your progress. Weighing yourself more frequently than that can lead to discouragement because weight fluctuates daily with changes in fluid balance.

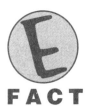

FACT

If you don't have someone to watch the baby while you exercise, then bring her with you. Walking is a great way to exercise! While at home, use baby's precious nap time to get in your exercise with a treadmill, exercise video, or other equipment.

Keeping a Food Diary

Food diaries can be a big help whether you are following a specific program or just trying to change some habits. A food diary can help increase your awareness of your eating habits and reinforce your education on the "good" foods to eat and the "good" way of eating. Putting your meals into writing makes a stronger impression in your mind and helps pinpoint the habits that may be undermining your attempts to lose weight. A food diary also helps you keep a written record of your commitment to eating balanced meals throughout the day. When keeping a food diary, it is important to follow some guidelines to make your effort as effective as possible. Write down everything you eat and drink, no matter how small you think it is. A handful of this and a nibble here all add up in the end! In addition, write down what you eat immediately afterwards. It is too easy to forget certain foods, like that candy bar you snuck in midday. Include the times that you ate meals and snacks, the type of food, and the exact amount you ate. Portion sizes can mean a lot, because the bigger the portion the more calories you eat.

Don't just use the diary for food you consume. Also use it to record your feelings as you eat throughout the day, such as boredom or stress. This helps you to realize why you are eating, which may not always be from hunger, and can help pinpoint food triggers. You can also record and keep track of your water intake and your daily exercise. The more you think about what you are eating, the more you can try to control what you are eating.

Setting Goals and Getting Motivated

Some women are eager to take off their pregnancy weight, while others may not be. It is important to lose the weight you gained throughout your pregnancy so you don't find yourself continually packing on the pounds. This can be a great time to set a goal to get to a healthy weight, especially if that wasn't the case before pregnancy. If you plan on becoming pregnant again down the road, you want to be at a healthy weight for a healthier pregnancy. Losing the extra weight can help you feel better; it can also make taking care of your newborn much less stressful.

Discover Your Motivations

Trying to change your lifestyle to a healthier one for better health and weight control can be difficult at times. It is important to have goals that you are working toward to keep you motivated! Before you start setting goals, it is important to identify what your motivation is and how ready you are to make needed lifestyle changes. It is helpful to assess your own motivation by asking yourself some of the following questions:

- What are my reasons for wanting to lose weight?
- Why is this important to me?
- What benefits do I expect to gain from losing weight?
- What would make this "worth it" to me?
- Is now the right time for me? Am I ready to make the commitment?

To help you stay motivated for the long haul, write down at least five important reasons you want to lose weight. Make them long-term goals, such as health and family, rather than short-term goals, such as a party next weekend. Put the sheet somewhere you can see it every day.

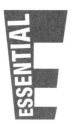

Get yourself motivated in any way that you can. Be creative, and use what works best for you! Do you sit in front of a computer all day long? Add a message to your screen saver to remind you of what you are trying to accomplish. You can put the message in code so only you know what it means. Every time you see it, it will remind you of what you should be doing!

Goal Setting: Now and Then

It is important to establish both short-term and long-term goals as part of your weight loss plan. Short-term goals help you reach long-term goals by initiating small steps and keeping you motivated throughout the process. Short-term goals can help change behaviors and/or keep you motivated. Your goals should deal with specific problems, such as the need to eat more vegetables, and should be specific about the what, where, when, and how of your planned changes. In other words, get yourself an action plan.

Short-term goals, such as drinking 64 ounces of water each day, can help change behaviors. Be specific about how you will reach your goal. It is too vague to simply say, "I will drink more water." This does not give you any specific action to work on. On the other hand, the statement, "I will buy a

32-ounce water bottle and fill it up and drink it twice a day" is specific enough that you can measure each day whether you have achieved your goal.

Short-term goals, such as a class reunion, can also help motivate you through your weight loss process, but make sure you line up another goal as soon as that event is over to keep you going. A specific event should not be your final or long-term goal. Make your long-term goals more than just weight loss. Make them goals that will emerge from the weight loss, such as getting healthy, defining a positive self-image, taking better care of your children, having more energy, improving the quality of your life, eating better, and enjoying physical activity.

One Step at a Time

Work on a few behaviors at a time, and once you have accomplished those, move on to a few more. Trying to bite off more than you can chew can be overwhelming as well as discouraging. Once you accomplish a short-term goal, move on to the next. A feeling of accomplishment can be a great motivational tool. Here's an example:

Long-Term Goal: Improve my health risk factors.
Short-Term Goal: Eat breakfast every day.
Action Plan: Buy healthy breakfast foods to have on hand, and get up fifteen minutes early to make time for breakfast.

Choosing a Commercial Weight-Loss Program

Weight loss is not as easy as it sounds for some people, who find they need some outside help. It is important to be aware of the different types of programs and options available so that you are able to make an informed choice. Do your homework before you sink your money into a program, and select a weight loss program that works for you. A responsible and safe weight-loss program should feature the following:

- The program should take into account your individual nutrient needs and supply your daily recommended levels of vitamins, minerals, and protein.

- The program should be moderate in calories (not too low) and should not leave out entire food groups.
- The program should encourage a safe, personalized physical activity program.
- The program should be directed toward a slow, steady weight loss of about ½ to 2 pounds per week and ½ to 1 pound if breastfeeding.
- If you are breastfeeding, the program should offer an eating plan especially for breastfeeding moms that is tailored to their special needs.
- The program should include plans for weight maintenance after the weight loss phase is over. Weight maintenance is the most difficult part of controlling weight and is not consistently implemented in weight-loss programs.
- The program should provide help in permanently changing your dietary as well as your exercise habits. The program should make changes to your previous lifestyle (before pregnancy) if that contributed to some of your weight gain.
- The program should provide behavior modification, including education in healthy eating habits and long-term plans to deal with weight problems.
- The program should provide you with a detailed disclosure of all fees and costs, including hidden fees for items such as special foods and supplements.

Most importantly, make sure the program is sensible and realistic. Make sure it is something you can (and will) stick with. You have a newborn at home now, so make sure the program fits your busy lifestyle, too.

Facing Fad Diets

No matter how eager you are to lose your pregnancy weight, fad diets are not the answer. Quicker and easy is not always better. That is doubly true for women who are breastfeeding and who need extra calories and nutrients for successful breastfeeding. There are hundreds of fad-type diet books and programs on the market today that lure people by promising quick and easy weight loss. These fad diets come and go quickly, with each one having a different twist: low fat, high carbohydrate; high fat, low carbohydrate; high protein; liquid supplements; food combining; eat for your blood type; and many others.

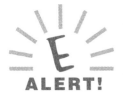

ALERT!

In general, fad diets have one thing in common—a point of restraint. Some of these restraints come in the form of carbohydrates; some are calories, specific foods, food groups, or fat. These restrictions can lead to severe nutritional deficiencies over time.

Fad diets do not touch on the emotional and behavioral ties that are associated with overeating, and they are usually so restrictive and unrealistic that most people can't stick with them very long. These diets do not help people establish healthful eating habits, and as a result many end up going back to old eating habits as soon as they are finished. Most people who use these diets end up gaining back most, if not more, of the weight they lost. This lays the foundation for an endless circle of diets without ever achieving successful long-term weight loss. This can cause a great deal of frustration, guilt, and feelings of failure.

Few fad diets encourage exercise, which is essential to losing weight and maintaining weight loss over a long period of time. Most people who lose weight and maintain weight successfully do not rely on a single strategy. In addition, many of these diet crazes are not backed up by scientific research and/or credible organizations. Your rule of thumb should be that if it sounds too good to be true, it probably is!

Is Your Weight Stuck?

Women will invariably experience intermittent plateaus while trying to lose their pregnancy weight. A weight-loss plateau is defined as a period of time during weight loss when your weight just won't move. The most important thing at this point is to not give up! Instead of blaming yourself, take a look at what you are eating and doing and use that energy to focus on problem solving. Plateaus can actually be a great learning opportunity for you.

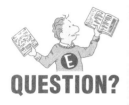

To break through a weight-loss plateau, should I eat fewer calories?
When you eat fewer than 800 or 1,000 calories a day, you body protects itself by turning down its thermostat to conserve every calorie it can get. Instead of decreasing your calorie intake, increase your exercise. You may need to re-evaluate your calorie needs. It's possible your body now needs fewer calories if you've lost a lot of weight and you have a smaller body size.

Why Me?

People hit weight-loss plateaus for a variety of reasons. You can hit a plateau because your body requires fewer calories to function as you lose weight, and your body may just need time to adjust. Or it may be that you have slowly started to adopt old habits again without even realizing it. Instead of getting down on yourself, remember the positive and successful changes that you have made to this point. Check out some of the following situations that could be problem areas, and start to problem-solve:

- Have your portion sizes increased? As you begin to lose weight, you may become less diligent about measuring portions. Go back to measuring your foods, and get back on track. A little extra food here and there is all your body may need to get stuck on a plateau.
- Are you doing the same amount of exercise you were doing when you began? If not, get yourself back on track.
- Has your exercise routine become too easy? Try something new! Step up to a more vigorous program, or just add a few more minutes.
- Do you do weight training as part of your exercise program? The more muscle you build, the more calories your body burns.
- Are you drinking enough water? Make sure you are getting at least eight 8-ounce glasses per day. Filling up on water during the day can make controlling your portion sizes easier at meals.
- Are late-night munchies or snacks getting out of hand? Continue to keep a food diary to help you pinpoint times when you may be letting your eating get out of control.

Appendix A

Dietary Guidelines for Americans

AIM FOR FITNESS

▶ Aim for a healthy weight.

Choose a lifestyle that combines sensible eating with regular physical activity. To be at your best, you need to avoid gaining weight, and many of us need to lose weight. Being overweight or obese increases your risk for high blood pressure, high blood cholesterol, heart disease, stroke, diabetes, certain types of cancer, arthritis, and breathing problems. A healthy weight is key to a long, healthy life.

▶ Be physically active each day.

Physical activity involves moving the body. A moderate physical activity is any activity that requires about as much energy as walking two miles in thirty minutes. Aim to accumulate at least thirty minutes (for adults) or sixty minutes (for children) of moderate physical activity most days of the week, preferably daily. If you already get thirty minutes of physical activity daily, you can gain even more health benefits by increasing the amount of time that you are physically active or by taking part in more vigorous activities. No matter what activity you choose, you can do it all at once, or spread it out over two or three episodes throughout the day.

BUILD A HEALTHY BASE

▶ Let the Food Guide Pyramid guide your food choices.

Different foods contain different nutrients and other healthful substances. No single food can supply all the nutrients in the amounts you need. For example, oranges provide vitamin C and folate but no vitamin B_{12}; cheese provides calcium and vitamin B_{12} but no vitamin C. To make sure you get all the nutrients and other substances you need for health, build a healthy base by using the Food Guide Pyramid as a starting point. Choose the recommended number of daily servings from each of the five major food groups.

▶ Choose a variety of grains daily, especially whole grains.

Foods made from grains (wheat, rice, and oats) help form the foundation of a nutritious diet. They provide vitamins, minerals, carbohydrates (starch and dietary fiber), and other substances that are important for good health. Grain products are low in fat, unless fat is added in processing, in preparation, or at the table. Whole grains differ from refined grains in the amount of fiber and nutrients they provide. Different whole-grain foods differ in nutrient content, so choose a variety of whole and enriched grains. Eating plenty of whole grains, such as whole-wheat bread or oatmeal as part of the healthful eating patterns described by these guidelines, may help protect you against many chronic diseases.

▶ Choose a variety of fruits and vegetables daily.

Fruits and vegetables are key parts of your daily diet. Eating plenty of fruits and vegetables of different kinds, as part of the healthful eating patterns described by these guidelines, may help protect you against many chronic diseases. It also promotes healthy bowel function. Fruits and vegetables provide essential vitamins and minerals, fiber, and other substances that are important for good health.

▶ Keep food safe to eat.

Foods that are safe from harmful bacteria, viruses, parasites, and chemical contaminants are vital for healthful eating. Safe means that the food poses little risk of foodborne illness. Farmers, food producers, markets, food-service establishments, and other food preparers have a role to keep food as safe as possible. However, we also need to keep and prepare foods safely in the home, and be alert when eating out.

CHOOSE SENSIBLY

▶ **Choose a diet that is low in saturated fat and cholesterol and moderate in total fat.**

Fats supply energy and essential fatty acids, and they help absorb carotenoids and the fat-soluble vitamins A, D, E, and K. You need some fat in the food you eat, but choose sensibly. Some kinds of fat, especially saturated fats, increase the risk for coronary heart disease by raising the blood cholesterol. In contrast, unsaturated fats (found mainly in vegetable oils) do not increase blood cholesterol. Fat intake in the United States as a proportion of total calories is lower than it was many years ago, but most people still eat too much saturated fat. Eating lots of fat of any type can provide excess calories.

▶ **Choose beverages and foods to moderate your intake of sugars.**

Sugars are carbohydrates and a source of energy (calories). Dietary carbohydrates also include the complex carbohydrates starch and dietary fiber. During digestion, all carbohydrates except fiber break down into sugars. Sugars and starches occur naturally in many foods that also supply other nutrients. Examples of these foods include milk, fruits, some vegetables, breads, cereals, and grains.

▶ **Choose and prepare foods with less salt.**

Many people can reduce their chances of developing high blood pressure by consuming less salt. Several other steps can also help keep your blood pressure in the healthy range. In the body, sodium, which you get mainly from salt, plays an essential role in regulating fluids and blood pressure. Many studies in diverse populations have shown that a high sodium intake is associated with higher blood pressure. There is no way to tell who might develop high blood pressure from eating too much salt. However, consuming less salt or sodium is not harmful and can be recommended for the healthy, normal person. At present, the firmest link between salt intake and health relates to blood pressure. High salt intake also increases the amount of calcium excreted in the urine. Eating less salt may decrease the loss of calcium from bone. Losing too much calcium from bone increases the risk of osteoporosis and bone fractures.

▶ **If you drink alcoholic beverages, do so in moderation.**

Alcoholic beverages supply calories but few nutrients. Alcoholic beverages are harmful when consumed in excess, and some people should not drink at all. Excess alcohol alters judgment and can lead to dependency and a great many other serious health problems. Taking more than one drink per day for women or two drinks per day for men can raise the risk for motor vehicle accidents and other injuries, as well as high blood pressure, stroke, violence, suicide, and certain types of cancer. Even one drink per day can slightly raise the risk of breast cancer. Alcohol consumption during pregnancy increases the risk of birth defects. Too much alcohol may cause social and psychological problems, cirrhosis of the liver, inflammation of the pancreas, and damage to the brain and heart. Heavy drinkers also are at risk of malnutrition because alcohol contains calories that may substitute for those in nutritious foods. If adults choose to drink alcoholic beverages, they should consume them only in moderation—and with meals to slow alcohol absorption.

The sixth edition of the *Dietary Guidelines for Americans* will be out in 2005. To find all updates refer to *www.usda.gov/cnpp*.

Source: *The Dietary Guidelines for Americans 2000*, 5th Edition (USDA and HHS).

Figuring Your Body Mass Index (BMI)

To figure out your BMI, use the following formula:

Weight (pounds) ÷ 2.2 = weight in kilograms (kg)
Height (inches) ÷ 39.37 = height in meters (m)
Weight (kg) ÷ height (m) squared = BMI

For example:
Sue weighs 165 pounds and is 5'6" or 66" tall:
165 pounds ÷ 2.2 = 75 kg
66" ÷ 39.37 = 1.68
75 kg ÷ (1.68 x 1.68) = 26.5 BMI

BMI Categories	
Underweight	less than 18.5
Normal weight	18.5 to 24.9
Overweight	25 to 29.9
Obesity	30 to 39.9 or greater
Severely Obese	greater than 40

Check your BMI against the following chart to see where your present weight places you for risk of health problems related to your body weight:

BMI	Risk for health problems related to body weight
20–25	Very low risk
26–30	Low risk
31–35	Moderate risk
36–39	High risk
40–plus	Very high risk

If your BMI is greater than 30, you should consult your personal physician for further evaluation, especially before becoming pregnant.

Appendix C

Additional Resources

Before, during, and after pregnancy, it is essential to know where to find sound nutrition information when you need it. The key is to use reputable and trustworthy sources. The information you read should not mislead you and should come from credible sources such as institutions, health professionals, journals, government organizations, and scientists. Before you take any type of nutritional or health advice from someone or something you read, consult a registered dietitian or doctor. The following is a list of associations and Web sites that will help you lead you to reliable nutrition and health information.

American Academy of Pediatrics

141 Northwest Point Boulevard
Elk Grove Village, IL 60007-1098
☎847-434-4000
✎www.aap.org

American College of Obstetricians and Gynecologists

409 12th St., S.W., P.O. Box 96920
Washington, D.C., 20090-6920
✎www.acog.org

American Dietetic Association

120 South Riverside Plaza, Suite 2000
Chicago, IL 60606-6995
☎800-877-1600
✎www.eatright.org

American Diabetes Association

ATTN: National Call Center
1701 North Beauregard Street
Alexandria, VA 22311
☎800-DIABETES (800-342-2383)
E-mail: AskADA@diabetes.org
✎www.diabetes.org

American Council on Exercise

4851 Paramount Drive
San Diego, California 92123
☎800-825-3636
✎www.acefitness.com

American Heart Association

National Center
7272 Greenville Ave.
Dallas, TX 75231
☎800-AHA-USA-1 (800-242-8721)
✎www.americanheart.org

American Lung Association

61 Broadway, 6th Floor
New York, NY 10006
☎1-800-LUNG-USA (800-586-4872)
✍*www.lungusa.org*

Environmental Protection Agency

Ariel Rios Building
1200 Pennsylvania Avenue, N.W.
Washington, D.C. 20460
☎202-272-0167
✍*www.epa.gov*

Food Allergy Network

Alletess Medical
216 Pleasant St.
Rockland, MA 02370
☎800-225-5404
E-mail: alletess@foodallergy.com
✍*www.foodallergy.com*

FDA (Food and Drug Administration)

5600 Fishers Lane
Rockville, MD 20857-0001
☎888-INFO-FDA (888-463-6332)
✍*www.fda.gov*

Food and Labeling Information

✍*www.cfsan.fda.gov*

Food and Nutrition Information Center

10301 Baltimore Avenue
Beltsville, MD 20705-2351
☎301-504-5719
E-mail: fnic@nal.usda.gov
✍*www.nal.usda.gov/fnic*

Institute of Medicine

The National Academies
2001 Wisconsin Ave., N.W.
Washington, D.C. 20007
E-mail: iomwww@nas.edu
✍*www.iom.edu*

National Eating Disorders Association

603 Stewart St., Suite 803
Seattle, WA 98101
☎206-382-3587
E-mail: info@nationaleatingdisorders.org
✍*www.nationaleatingdisorders.org*

National Institutes of Health

9000 Rockville Pike
Bethesda, MD 20892
☎301-496-4000
✍*www.nih.gov*

U.S. Department of Health and Human Services

200 Independence Ave., S.W.
Washington, D.C. 20201
☎877-696-6775
E-mail: HHS.mail@hhs.gov
✍*www.dhhs.gov*

Visit the following Web sites for more information on vegetarianism:

The Vegetarian Resource Group
www.vrg.org

Vegetarian Times
www.vegetariantimes.com

North American Vegetarian Society
www.navs-online.org

Vegsource.com
www.vegsource.com

Vegan Action
www.vegan.org

Visit the following Web sites for more information on soy products:

U.S. Soyfoods Directory
www.soyfoods.com

Talksoy.com
www.talksoy.com

Soybean.org
www.soybean.org

United Soybean Board
www.unitedsoybean.org

Visit the following Web sites for more information on health and pregnancy:

WebMD.com
www.webmd.com

HealthFinder
www.healthfinder.gov

American Pregnancy Association
www.americanpregnancy.org

ParentsPlace.com
www.parentsplace.com

FitPregnancy
www.fitpregnancy.com

Kids' Health for Parents
www.kidhealth.org

The National Woman's Health Information Center
www.4woman.gov

Pregnancy.org
www.pregnancy.org

Index

THE EVERYTHING SERIES!

BUSINESS

Everything® Business Planning Book
Everything® Coaching and Mentoring Book
Everything® Fundraising Book
Everything® Home-Based Business Book
Everything® Landlording Book
Everything® Leadership Book
Everything® Managing People Book
Everything® Negotiating Book
Everything® Online Business Book
Everything® Project Management Book
Everything® Robert's Rules Book, $7.95
Everything® Selling Book
Everything® Start Your Own Business Book
Everything® Time Management Book

COMPUTERS

Everything® Computer Book

COOKBOOKS

Everything® Barbecue Cookbook
Everything® Bartender's Book, $9.95
Everything® Chinese Cookbook
Everything® Chocolate Cookbook
Everything® Cookbook
Everything® Dessert Cookbook
Everything® Diabetes Cookbook
Everything® Fondue Cookbook
Everything® Grilling Cookbook
Everything® Holiday Cookbook
Everything® Indian Cookbook
Everything® Low-Carb Cookbook
Everything® Low-Fat High-Flavor Cookbook
Everything® Low-Salt Cookbook
Everything® Mediterranean Cookbook
Everything® Mexican Cookbook
Everything® One-Pot Cookbook
Everything® Pasta Cookbook
Everything® Quick Meals Cookbook
Everything® Slow Cooker Cookbook
Everything® Soup Cookbook

Everything® Thai Cookbook
Everything® Vegetarian Cookbook
Everything® Wine Book

HEALTH

Everything® Alzheimer's Book
Everything® Anti-Aging Book
Everything® Diabetes Book
Everything® Dieting Book
Everything® Hypnosis Book
Everything® Low Cholesterol Book
Everything® Massage Book
Everything® Menopause Book
Everything® Nutrition Book
Everything® Reflexology Book
Everything® Reiki Book
Everything® Stress Management Book
Everything® Vitamins, Minerals, and
          Nutritional Supplements Book

HISTORY

Everything® American Government Book
Everything® American History Book
Everything® Civil War Book
Everything® Irish History & Heritage Book
Everything® Mafia Book
Everything® Middle East Book

HOBBIES & GAMES

Everything® Bridge Book
Everything® Candlemaking Book
Everything® Card Games Book
Everything® Cartooning Book
Everything® Casino Gambling Book, 2nd Ed.
Everything® Chess Basics Book
Everything® Crossword and Puzzle Book
Everything® Crossword Challenge Book
Everything® Drawing Book
Everything® Digital Photography Book
Everything® Easy Crosswords Book
Everything® Family Tree Book

Everything® Games Book
Everything® Knitting Book
Everything® Magic Book
Everything® Motorcycle Book
Everything® Online Genealogy Book
Everything® Photography Book
Everything® Poker Strategy Book
Everything® Pool & Billiards Book
Everything® Quilting Book
Everything® Scrapbooking Book
Everything® Sewing Book
Everything® Soapmaking Book

HOME IMPROVEMENT

Everything® Feng Shui Book
Everything® Feng Shui Decluttering Book, $9.95
Everything® Fix-It Book
Everything® Homebuilding Book
Everything® Home Decorating Book
Everything® Landscaping Book
Everything® Lawn Care Book
Everything® Organize Your Home Book

EVERYTHING® KIDS' BOOKS

All titles are $6.95

Everything® Kids' Baseball Book, 3rd Ed.
Everything® Kids' Bible Trivia Book
Everything® Kids' Bugs Book
Everything® Kids' Christmas Puzzle
          & Activity Book
Everything® Kids' Cookbook
Everything® Kids' Halloween Puzzle
          & Activity Book
Everything® Kids' Hidden Pictures Book
          Everything® Kids' Joke Book
Everything® Kids' Knock Knock Book
Everything® Kids' Math Puzzles Book
Everything® Kids' Mazes Book
Everything® Kids' Money Book

All Everything® books are priced at $12.95 or $14.95, unless otherwise stated. Prices subject to change without notice.

Everything® Kids' Monsters Book
Everything® Kids' Nature Book
Everything® Kids' Puzzle Book
Everything® Kids' Riddles & Brain Teasers Book
Everything® Kids' Science Experiments Book
Everything® Kids' Soccer Book
Everything® Kids' Travel Activity Book

KIDS' STORY BOOKS

Everything® Bedtime Story Book
Everything® Bible Stories Book
Everything® Fairy Tales Book

LANGUAGE

Everything® Conversational Japanese Book
    (with CD), $19.95
Everything® Inglés Book
Everything® French Phrase Book, $9.95
Everything® Learning French Book
Everything® Learning German Book
Everything® Learning Italian Book
Everything® Learning Latin Book
Everything® Learning Spanish Book
Everything® Sign Language Book
Everything® Spanish Phrase Book, $9.95
Everything® Spanish Verb Book, $9.95

MUSIC

Everything® Drums Book (with CD), $19.95
Everything® Guitar Book
Everything® Home Recording Book
Everything® Playing Piano and Keyboards Book
Everything® Rock & Blues Guitar Book
    (with CD), $19.95
Everything® Songwriting Book

NEW AGE

Everything® Astrology Book
Everything® Dreams Book
Everything® Ghost Book
Everything® Love Signs Book, $9.95
Everything® Meditation Book
Everything® Numerology Book
Everything® Paganism Book
Everything® Palmistry Book
Everything® Psychic Book
Everything® Spells & Charms Book
Everything® Tarot Book
Everything® Wicca and Witchcraft Book

PARENTING

Everything® Baby Names Book
Everything® Baby Shower Book
Everything® Baby's First Food Book
Everything® Baby's First Year Book
Everything® Birthing Book
Everything® Breastfeeding Book
Everything® Father-to-Be Book
Everything® Get Ready for Baby Book
Everything® Getting Pregnant Book
Everything® Homeschooling Book
Everything® Parent's Guide to Children
    with Asperger's Syndrome
Everything® Parent's Guide to Children
    with Autism
Everything® Parent's Guide to Children
    with Dyslexia
Everything® Parent's Guide to Positive Discipline
Everything® Parent's Guide to Raising a
    Successful Child
Everything® Parenting a Teenager Book
Everything® Potty Training Book, $9.95
Everything® Pregnancy Book, 2nd Ed.
Everything® Pregnancy Fitness Book
Everything® Pregnancy Nutrition Book
Everything® Pregnancy Organizer, $15.00
Everything® Toddler Book
Everything® Tween Book

PERSONAL FINANCE

Everything® Budgeting Book
Everything® Get Out of Debt Book
Everything® Homebuying Book, 2nd Ed.
Everything® Homeselling Book
Everything® Investing Book
Everything® Online Business Book
Everything® Personal Finance Book
Everything® Personal Finance in Your
    20s & 30s Book
Everything® Real Estate Investing Book
Everything® Wills & Estate Planning Book

PETS

Everything® Cat Book
Everything® Dog Book
Everything® Dog Training and Tricks Book
Everything® Golden Retriever Book
Everything® Horse Book
Everything® Labrador Retriever Book
Everything® Poodle Book

Everything® Puppy Book
Everything® Rottweiler Book
Everything® Tropical Fish Book

REFERENCE

Everything® Car Care Book
Everything® Classical Mythology Book
Everything® Einstein Book
Everything® Etiquette Book
Everything® Great Thinkers Book
Everything® Philosophy Book
Everything® Psychology Book
Everything® Shakespeare Book
Everything® Toasts Book

RELIGION

Everything® Angels Book
Everything® Bible Book
Everything® Buddhism Book
Everything® Catholicism Book
Everything® Christianity Book
Everything® Jewish History & Heritage Book
Everything® Judaism Book
Everything® Koran Book
Everything® Prayer Book
Everything® Saints Book
Everything® Understanding Islam Book
Everything® World's Religions Book
Everything® Zen Book

SCHOOL & CAREERS

Everything® After College Book
Everything® Alternative Careers Book
Everything® College Survival Book
Everything® Cover Letter Book
Everything® Get-a-Job Book
Everything® Job Interview Book
Everything® New Teacher Book
Everything® Online Job Search Book
Everything® Personal Finance Book
Everything® Practice Interview Book
Everything® Resume Book, 2nd Ed.
Everything® Study Book

SELF-HELP/
RELATIONSHIPS

Everything® Dating Book
Everything® Divorce Book
Everything® Great Sex Book

All Everything® books are priced at $12.95 or $14.95, unless otherwise stated. Prices subject to change without notice.

Everything® Kama Sutra Book
Everything® Self-Esteem Book

SPORTS & FITNESS

Everything® Body Shaping Book
Everything® Fishing Book
Everything® Fly-Fishing Book
Everything® Golf Book
Everything® Golf Instruction Book
Everything® Knots Book
Everything® Pilates Book
Everything® Running Book
Everything® T'ai Chi and QiGong Book
Everything® Total Fitness Book
Everything® Weight Training Book
Everything® Yoga Book

TRAVEL

Everything® Family Guide to Hawaii
Everything® Family Guide to New York City,
     2nd Ed.

Everything® Family Guide to Washington D.C.,
     2nd Ed.
Everything® Family Guide to the Walt Disney
     World Resort®, Universal Studios®,
     and Greater Orlando, 4th Ed.
Everything® Guide to Las Vegas
Everything® Guide to New England
Everything® Travel Guide to the Disneyland
     Resort®, California Adventure®,
     Universal Studios®, and the
     Anaheim Area

WEDDINGS

Everything® Bachelorette Party Book, $9.95
Everything® Bridesmaid Book, $9.95
Everything® Creative Wedding Ideas Book
Everything® Elopement Book, $9.95
Everything® Father of the Bride Book, $9.95
Everything® Groom Book, $9.95
Everything® Jewish Wedding Book
Everything® Mother of the Bride Book, $9.95
Everything® Wedding Book, 3rd Ed.

Everything® Wedding Checklist, $7.95
Everything® Wedding Etiquette Book, $7.95
Everything® Wedding Organizer, $15.00
Everything® Wedding Shower Book, $7.95
Everything® Wedding Vows Book, $7.95
Everything® Weddings on a Budget Book, $9.95

WRITING

Everything® Creative Writing Book
Everything® Get Published Book
Everything® Grammar and Style Book
Everything® Grant Writing Book
Everything® Guide to Writing a Novel
Everything® Guide to Writing Children's Books
Everything® Screenwriting Book
Everything® Writing Well Book

Introducing an exceptional new line of beginner craft books from the *Everything*® series!

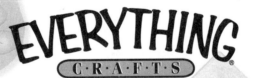

EVERYTHING
C·R·A·F·T·S®

All titles are $14.95.

Everything® Crafts—Create Your Own Greeting Cards
1-59337-226-4
Everything® Crafts—Polymer Clay for Beginners
1-59337-230-2

Everything® Crafts—Rubberstamping Made Easy
1-59337-229-9
Everything® Crafts—Wedding Decorations
and Keepsakes
1-59337-227-2

Available wherever books are sold!
To order, call 800-872-5627, or visit us at *www.everything.com*
Everything® and everything.com® are registered trademarks of F+W Publications, Inc.